A Safer Death

Multidisciplinary Aspects of Terminal Care

A Safer Death

Multidisciplinary Aspects of Terminal Care

Edited by
Anne Gilmore
Prince and Princess of Wales Hospice
Glasgow, Scotland

and
Stan Gilmore
Stirling University
Stirling, Scotland

Plenum Press • New York and London

Library of Congress Cataloging in Publication Data

International Conference of the Prince and Princess of Wales Hospice on Multidisciplinary Aspects of Terminal Care (1st: 1987: Glasgow, Strathclyde)
    A safer death.

    "Proceedings of the First International Conference of the Prince and Princess of
Wales Hospice on Multidisciplinary Aspects of Terminal Care, held September 8–10,
1987, in Glasgow, Scotland" — T.p. verso.
    1. Terminal care — Congresses. 2. Terminal care — Psychological aspects — Congress-
es. I. Gilmore, Anne. II. Gilmore, Stan. III. Title.
R726.8.I56   1987   362.1′75   88-12414
ISBN-13: 978-1-4615-8361-5   e-ISBN-13: 978-1-4615-8359-2
DOI: 10.1007/978-1-4615-8359-2

Proceedings of the First International Conference of the Prince and Princess
of Wales Hospice on Multidisciplinary Aspects of Terminal Care,
held September 8–10, 1987, in Glasgow, Scotland.

© 1988 Plenum Press, New York
Softcover reprint of the hardcover 1st edition 1988

A Division of Plenum Publishing Corporation
233 Spring Street, New York, N.Y. 10013

PREFACE

During the past two decades professional interest in Terminal Care has increased dramatically. It is always difficult to trace the origins of a change of emphasis in medical and nursing care but it is likely that three influences have contributed to bring this about. Firstly, the rise of the modern hospice movement with its recognition that dying and mourning are normal life events and that the lay person has a role in these events no less important than the health professional; secondly, the development of sophisticated and successful techniques of palliative care and pain control; and lastly, the increasing expectations of the populace in advanced countries for a comprehensive and sensitive service for patients, family and care givers at the terminal phase of illness.

It is significant that these developments in the care and management of the terminally ill are not confined either to one country or the sole prerogative of a single discipline. This is reflected in the papers collected in this volume which were originally presented at the International Conference on Multidisciplinary Aspects of Terminal Care organised by The Prince and Princess of Wales Hospice in Glasgow, Scotland, U.K.

The cross-fertilisation of ideas, experiences, and assessments provided by the contributors in a multicultural and multidisciplinary context presented in this volume will be found stimulating and inspirational for both the professional and the lay person in the care of the dying.

Michael Bond
Vice Principal and Professor
of Psychological Medicine
University of Glasgow
Scotland, U.K.   1988

CONTENTS

PART ONE

PROBLEMS OF DEATH AND DYING

"SAFE DEATH" IN THE POSTMODERN WORLD

Robert Kastenbaum

Arizona State University
Tempe, Arizona, USA

SOME DEATHS ARE BETTER THAN OTHERS

Let us begin with the proposition that some deaths are better than others. A student of logic would make mince pie of this statement in no time. "You are indulging in a lazy, gross, and elementary error! Dying is not death. People may die in a thousand ways. This does not mean that there are a thousand kinds of death. "Dying" is our word for the particular way a person lives as life approaches cessation. "Death" is the word for our ignorance regarding what happens - or does not happen - when people stop living and dying. We may have our preferences for modalities of dying, but all reach the same destination."

These points are well taken. But logic does not often stand in the way of our fondest or most fearful endeavours. Perhaps it is because we are so ignorant of death; perhaps it is because our minds cannot fasten securely on a state - or non-state - that seems so radically different from the usual categories and contents of our mental life. Or perhaps it is because the experiences and circumstances that precede death arouse so great a concern that we are absorbed by what we can observe and interpret on life's stage, rather than by what we can only wonder might be concealed from our view in the wings.

Generally, when we encounter such concepts as the "good death" or the "appropriate death", it is actually the last phase of life that is at issue. And it is this issue that is at the core of hospice. "Prince and Princess of Wales Hospice: Purveyor of Fine Deaths" is an emblem I have not seen, but it is likely to be an expectation nevertheless. Expectation! This is a concept whose importance is difficult to overestimate. How hospice is judged and how hospice judges itself depends not only on what happens but on the relationship between what happens and what we expect, hope, fear, and fantasize.

It becomes important, then, to examine the criteria that are applied to evaluate "better" and "worse" deaths - or, if we don't mind sounding awkward, "better or worse dyings". The observations I will be sharing with you come from a variety of clinical experiences and research projects, with an emphasis on those in which I have been directly involved myself. But first I must tell you of a conversation that occurred at an international conference not so many years ago. All the participants in this

3

discussion group were active as service providers and researchers: you would recognise most of the names. Suddenly, one of the participants stunned the group with an outburst of fury - not disagreement, not anger - fury. We were fools at a conference of fools. The new enlightenment about death, even the hospice movement itself, this was all the cruelest imaginable nonsense. And then, he started to weep. Why the fury, why the tears? This man, a physician, had our admiration and respect for the humane care he provided to children who suffered from life threatening diseases. He was capable, mature, courageous, a model of strength in this difficult field.

He could and did explain after the fury and with the tears still in his eyes. One of his young patients had died recently - and died a "bad death". Despite everything that he and his staff could do, the youngster "bled out". The scene was horrifying to the family and to the professional care-givers as well. They had worked so hard and so resourcefully to help this child feel comfortable and enjoy what was left of life. But the final scene had come at the wrong time and the wrong place and in the wrong way. As we listened to his account we realised that in his own way he probably felt the pain of the "bad death" as acutely and deeply as the child's own parents. This pain had turned into fury because crucial expectations had been dashed. Here they had been, health care professionals with state of the art knowledge, with compassion, and with the full involvement of family members - and the death had been traumatic to them all. "I couldn't sit here another minute and hear all this talk about hospice goals, about spirituality, about serenity - damn it! We couldn't even stop the damn bleeding!"

A few years after this poignant and revealing incident took place, I could not help but notice that expectations for the "good death" were continuing to rise. In the United States there was a spate of articles, books, workshops, and television programmes that portrayed the last phase of life as a glorious experience. Dying was pretty wonderful - or it should be pretty wonderful. It was not enough to be relatively free of pain, nausea, and other distressing symptoms. It was not enough to remain in close contact with one's most cherished and supportive intimates. One had the right to expect more. The death bed scene was to be a peak experience, a fulfillment, a transcendental passage. Precisely how and why this expectation captured so many minds is a fascinating topic that must be left aside for the moment. The alarming point was that society was now generating expectations and fantasies that could be met, only on rare occasions, if at all. Dedicated professionals and devoted family members might provide superb care - and yet the death might be judged as "not good enough" when compared with the unchecked fantasies. At this point in time there was the danger that hospice could never keep up with the fantasies. And how much more devastating it would be in those unfortunate circumstances when the best available care could not even guarantee a death bed scene free of distress. "We couldn't even stop the damn bleeding!"

It seemed to me about a decade ago that we had two levels of fantasy with which to contend. The foundation level was built upon the expectation that one could pass from life to death with little distress, fuss, and inconvenience. I classified this type of expectation as "healthy dying" (Kastenbaum, 1979). We the people of the United States were now willing to acknowledge the fact of mortality - but only "on condition". This condition was that we should die in good health. The second level was even more ambitious. Dying should be somehow better than living - more meaningful, more spiritual, more ennobling, and perhaps, more enjoyable as well. Popular books and movies such as Love Story presented this fantasy in a form that appealed to a great many people.

Here are some of the specific hopes and expectations for the "good death", as drawn from clinical and research observations. I must caution

4

that these will seem confusing unless we pay strict attention to the frame of reference. Whether a situation is perceived as appropriate or outrageous, comforting or threatening, meaningful or meaningless depends on the perceiver as much as the situation.

If at all possible, the dying person should be an elderly adult. Almost all of the "worst deaths" have involved children and young adults; almost all of the "best deaths" have been those of old men and women who were "released from their suffering" or quietly "slipped away" without any bother.

Perhaps you do not agree with these statements. You are not obliged to agree with these statements. These, however, faithfully summarise what many caregivers believe to be true; it is the way they have interpreted and judged their own experiences. This is not everybody's perspective; but it is the perspective of many caregivers who have been required to work with terminally ill patients in traditional medical settings without any special education, training, or preparation. Perhaps you suspect that these judg- ments have been influenced rather too much by their own values and fears. Young people are supposed to live and thrive; the old are supposed to die. Perhaps you have noticed that the death of a young person threatens a comforting illusion while the death of an old person tends to reinforce the same illusion, namely, that the Catcher of Souls obeys a set of implicit regulations. Death is just doing his job when he harvests the old; every- body else has claim to a certain degree of immunity. I would agree with these suspicions. They are confirmed, for example, every time a caregiver simply assumes that a sick and vulnerable old person is ready for death and makes sure to perpetuate this belief by avoiding intimate, mind-to-mind contact. What if the old lady is really full of life and no more eager to die than the young boy? It's best not to expose ourselves to possibilities so discordant with our fixed assumptions and cherished illusions.

Here is another component of the "better death."

The relatively acceptable death is the one that nobody notices.

Once again, the perspective involved is that of people who have absorbed assumptions, stereotypes, and customs from their societies, adding their own individual anxieties. It is a perspective held in common by many lay people as well as professional caregivers, and was especially prevalent in the pre-hospice era. In the ideal situation, the dying person is drugged, sleeping, or comatose and therefore passes blankly from unawareness to oblivion. Nobody else is required to notice the passing - it doesn't happen on my floor or my shift, and, if it does, really nothing has happened at all. We simply initiate the postmortem routine. The false-bottomed stretcher that is wheeled through the back corridors of a world famous hospital, bearing a hidden corpse, is a characteristic part of this process. The ideal of transforming the passage from life to death into a non-event was later overtaken by the headier fantasies that have already been mentioned, but we still encounter people who are convinced that hear no dying, see no dying, feel no dying is the non-consummation most devoutly to be desired.

Here is a very different version of the "better death":

The good death is the one we face in an alert, composed state of mind with the opportunity to bid farewell to life and our loved ones in our own way.

This view is obviously quite different from that which prefers dying to pass unnoticed by everyone involved. Unfortunately, it is not unusual for these views to collide. Two competing visions of the acceptable death may create additional stress, tension, even tragedy. Either the dying person or a caregiver may hold either view, and both may fail to explicitly recognise their differences, let alone reconcile them.

Side results from the National Hospice Demonstration Study may be helpful here. This large scale study was chiefly concerned with determining if hospices in the United States were, in fact, performing in accordance with their stated principles, how patient and family outcomes compared with traditional care, and whether or not there was a cost savings involved (Mor et al., in press). But we also had the opportunity to explore a little of the patient's own views and preferences - a much too limited exploration, unfortunately. We asked some of these terminally ill cancer patients what they would like to have happen during the last three days of their lives. There was one particular pattern of response that emphasised mental alertness and control. These men and women hoped to play a central role in their own exit scenes. For them, it would be unacceptable, frightening, disappointing to feel themselves in a mental haze and to have others make all the moves. Their last days were to be days of living.

Before we rush to conclusions, however, consider one additional fact. It was only about one person in 20 who held this view. The great majority of these patients whose death was in near prospect did not attach that much importance to mental alertness and control. It was not a crucial priority for them. Consider what might occur, then, in the terminal care situation. A key service provider might hold the somewhat heroic conception that it is best to be fully alert in the face of death, with all other aspects being secondary. This view would accord very well with a few patients and, together, they might achieve their consensual goal. But in many more instances, the service provider's underlying vision of clear-eyed, heroic passage might create tensions and pressures for the patient. Further more, the opposite state of affairs could also generate serious difficulties. The service provider who emphasises passive comforting may often be acting in a manner consistent with the patient's own wishes - but every now and again this will have a catastrophic effect on the person for whom awareness and autonomy remain of the highest priority. It is not simply that we may have different visions of the good or acceptable death that these visions have the potential to collide with each other in crucial situations.

Here is still another version of the "good death."

The good death occurs within the context of ordinary life.

This view finds a middle ground between the denial and resistance of the "death nobody notices" and the heroic stand of those who intend to look Death in the eye. If I may refer again to some of the side results of the National Hospice Demonstration Study, it would appear that there are many who hold this middle ground. Most often it is the mature, family-orientated adult who hopes that life will continue in something resembling its familiar routine until the end comes. In fact, this was the most common view expressed by the terminally ill cancer patients who participated in the study. They knew the world, themselves, and their illness too well to expect death-bed miracles. What they sought was a sense of security and belongingness with the people who had mattered most to them through the years. Fortunately, the overall results of the National Hospice Demonstration Study indicated that this hope was often fulfilled. Those who had selected the hospice alternative were more likely to end their lives with their loved ones at home. There is obviously a good match between the expectations of older adults who have lived for some time with their illness and the resources available to hospice organisations. However, as we will see in a moment, it might be a mistake to assume that hospice philosophy and practice will continue to be so well matched with those whose deaths are in near prospect.

By contrast, here is still another perspective on the "good death" –

The "good death" is the quick, cost-efficient, no risk death.

You will recogise immediately that this is the perspective of the bureaucrat, the budget manager, the legal advisor. At a physical and emotional distance from the dying person, family, and caregivers, the bureaucrat has his own set of priorities. We often see this perspective at work in the United States. A terminally ill patient who may yet live "too long" or "too expensively" may become the pawn of bureaucratic chess players who want to remove this fiscally unsound person from their own account books. Similarly, the goal of avoiding malpractice suits may take precedence over clinical and humanistic considerations. Whatever we may think of the bureaucratic perspective, it is too influential to ignore, at least in the United States. The visions of a "good" or "acceptable" death that are held by the patient, family, and caregivers often must compete with the cost-efficient orientation of the bureaucrat.

Here is still another version of the "good death" that might not meet with everybody's approval –

The "good death" is the one we choose to produce.

This is the intentioned death that presents itself to the hunter or sniper's gunsight. This is the intentioned death by which slaughterhouse operators earn their profit. This is the sporting death, the vengeful death, the profitable death, and also the death that brings relief and delight whenever a human, himself scared to death, turns killer.

It might appear not only inappropriate, but in bad taste, to mention on this occasion some of the ways in which, as individuals and as a society, we choose to kill. However, the same societies that attempt to prevent and cure illness and to comfort the dying have also devoted themselves to killing with no less enthusiasm. We indulge in the expensive luxury of neglect and evasion if we do not face the fact that death at times thrills, fascinates, and motivates us – especially if we can have our own hands on the trigger, rather than our images in the gunsight.

There is at least one other aspect of the "good death" that must be considered. It is this aspect that will take us directly into the topic of "safe death" and the emerging challenge to hospice and society.

The "good death" is the product of the right kind of disease. Actually, the converse proposition is more to the point: the "bad death" is the product of the wrong kind of disease – wrong for any number of reasons, but, most fundamentally, wrong because it punctures some of our most sustaining hopes and illusions.

Let us turn now to some of the attitudes and meanings that have become associated with specific causes of death. If this requires a little attention to the past, please be assured that the intention is to help put the present and future into perspective.

WHEN DEATH TAKES CATASTROPHIC SHAPES

History provides us with some examples of deaths that many people could face – face with courage, resignation, or even longing and excitement. There is little doubt that death on the field of honorable warfare was viewed as acceptable by the fighting men of many cultures. This is not to say that the warriors preferred death to survival, although there was instances in which this attitude was observed. Honorable death in battle and suicide when honor was at stake were among the types of death that could be faced with courage or equanimity. A larger number of deaths seemed to call forth an attitude of resignation or fatalism. Worn down by illness and stress, deprived of adequate nutrician, weak and increasingly helpless, people nameless to the future died quietly. Deaths by exhaustion, malnutrition, injury, and infection were commonplace. There was suffering and distress, but at times there were also rituals and fantasies to soften the blow. It is clear, I think, that many people could cope with dying and the prospect of death. It was the expected end to a life that had often been hard and painful, and so was not out of keeping with the character of that life itself.

But death has sometimes taken a more horrendous shape. We speak now of something beyond the simple cessation of life and its attendant distress. Horrendous death threatens the values, the meanings, the very stuff that gives coherence to the world and one's own self. It may even take the form of an "anti-self", an adversary and antithesis that represents one's own characteristics but in an inverted, distorted, and frightening manner. If there is a "normal" death that can be compared with "normal sleep", then horrendous death must be likened to the nocturnal terrors of the nightmare.

When we awaken from a nightmare, there is a tendency to laugh with relief. Similarly, there is a tendency for people to treat some of the most extravagant terrors of earlier generations as material suitable for parody. A prime example is the first type of horrendous death that I call - or recall - to your attention. Your imagination is required because imagination is almost always the home for this type of death. The probable fact that this kind of death is very uncommon in "real life" has not made it any less compelling to the susceptible mind.

Imagine, if you will a darkness deeper than the night. Our eyes, hands, and feet are almost useless as protection. On the reality level, we might be medieval peasants hurrying to reach home before a pack of wolves emerges from the gathering darkness. However, we might also be living at almost any time and place in human history and experiencing fantasies that are even more intense than fear of an actual encounter with an actual beast. I must describe this form of horrendous death at two levels of psychological impact. At the physical and sensory level we imagine an attack by an overpowerful, foul-smelling, merciless creature that, for all its appalling characteristics, nevertheless reminds us uncomfortably of ourselves. This creature stinks of death, yet there is also a crazed sexual component as well. At different periods of history we might have whispered different names for this beast from the darkness, this Seth, this Typhoeus, this Lucifer, this Beserker, this Vampire. Whatever the name, it has always wanted our blood. Both our life and our death then became its possession.

At the level of deeper resonances, this form of horrendous death is the personification of our own most unacceptable impulses and fears. It is an encounter with The Other - that is to say, with an alternative self that seeks our mind, body, and blood for purposes our respectable, law-abiding personalities never would condone. In olden days this vision of terror was associated with primitive fears of a death-god arising from the earth itself. Later the Catholic Church would overlay this terror with sharp distinctions between light and dark, God and Devil, the saved and the damned. One aspect has been noted recently in an historical study by Patricia Ann Yeomans who writes that "In many ways, the church equated the vampire with evil, defined it as such, and through excommunication assured the existence of restless souls - those who had not been buried on hallowed ground, a ready-made regiment of the damned. The church representatives were also the exterminators of the vampire, responsible for hunting down, stalking, and burning their bloated corpses. This created a huge well in the imagination where the vampire took shape, a horrible bloodthirsty monster with all the powers of Satan himself" (Yeomans, 1986).

This split between our day-selves and the midnight monsters of our imagination seems quite out of keeping with the postmodern world where our tool has become the computer rather than the plow, and our fears center on high-tech megadeath rather than bloodthirsty monsters. In fact, one might think that what at times stimulated authentic terror in the past is well utilised now as material for cheap horror films - and even these now tend to parody their own subject matter.

This is what one might think. We may need to think again, however, and will do so after we have reminded ourselves of several other varieties of catastrophic death.

History reveals that the so-called Black Death not only took an enormous toll of human life but also made a powerful impression that retained some of its power for many years afterward. Recent studies have suggested that most of the casualties were caused not by the bubonic plague, as so long believed, but by anthrax, a disease most often associated with sheep and cattle (Twigg, 1984). Whatever the medical cause, however, the effects on the individual mind and social customs were significant and widespread, ranging from childhood games to artistic expression. I would call your attention to a few of these consequences that are most relevant for us today. The sudden onset of this agonising and disfiguring illness was often interpreted as divine retribution. We ourselves have sinned against God, or there are those among us who have aroused divine wrath. The victim most often had seen others die in agony and despair and had noted that death's handiwork - decomposition - seemed to begin even while life remained. There was time, then, to develop the most alarming state of apprehension before one's own turn came. It is likely that fears of a death too painful, too disfiguring, too invasive that were stimulated by the Black Death have been passed along through the generations, reinforced now and again by other incidents.

This shape of catastrophic death, then, could seem beyond human endurance: we had been rejected by God, and abandoned to pain and disfigurement against which ordinary reason and resolution seemed inadequate. Furthermore, the professional caregivers, such as they were, as well as the church authorities, could not be counted upon to provide comfort. The victim was alone with raw death, or, as Phillippe Aries (1981) might say, with untamed death. Again, we will return in a moment to this particular nightmare form of dying.

There are many causes of death, and always have been. Some of these modalities, however, have exercised an especially strong influence on our minds. May I remind you, very briefly, of a few more life threatening conditions that constitute part of the historical background against which hospice and its particular mission has arisen.

Soon after European voyagers found the New World, a new disease made its appearance and became a scourge everywhere: the "French Disease", the "English Disease", the "German Disease", and the "Neopolitan Disease" were all, of course, syphilis. Many people considered to have "leprosy" were also syphilics. Some of the associations that haunt syphilis today were generated during a more recent period of time. A major outbreak of syphilis occurred in Eastern Europe soon after World War I. This epidemic with its many deaths took place among people who lived in unstable, overcrowded, and grossly unhygienic circumstances. The idea that syphilis is "dirty", and brings us a particularly "dirty" death owes something to the havoc this disease has wrought to displaced and oppressed populations. An even more consistent theme, however, is the undeniable link with sexuality: the deterioration and death that could be regarded as the "wages of sin". Syphilis brings us the immoral death. But the association cuts even deeper and wider. Men would frequent prostitutes and then infect their own wives who, in turn, might bear children who were also afflicted with the disease. The intimacy and pleasure of sexual relations became threatened by both the reality and the fear of syphilis. And it was within this context of dread and suspicion that procreation had to proceed. There was no way to conceive a child without taking some risk - most often, the burden of the risk being placed on the woman. Romantic intimacy, sexual relations, and procreation were all threatened, then, by a disease that might not only take one's life, but also stain one's reputation and self-concept.

Notice, if you will, how two other life threatening diseases have given rise to different orientations to death. If our life is not in the blood, then it is in our breath. The belief that life enters and leaves through the breath is one of the most ancient ideas known to humankind. Tuberculosis literally took our breath away. In the nineteenth century, the struggle for breath became emblematic of the death bed scene, with tuberculosis as the primary model. From the observer's standpoint - that is, from the standpoint of somebody who might later become a victim - tuberculosis was alarming for its production of a wasted body and sunken eyes. The living person had started to resemble death. One hesitated to approach even a loved one who coughed so ominously, who lost blood through nose and mouth, and whose death seemed ready to spring forth and attack its next victim. The fact that tuberculosis so often claimed the young was especially distressing.

From this death that claimed our very breath, society tried to construct a more positive, compensating image. If the bright and talented are taken young, and if their eyes shine bright with fever, then there must be a special genius that presides over their deaths. The idea that mental life becomes enhanced as death approaches did have some occasional basis in reality. Largely, however, it was a compensatory vision that focused on young people falling to tuberculosis. Perhaps the tragedy of premature death had been somehow moderated through its romantic transformation.

The other vision of death I wish to select from history is of the type that makes the skin crawl and chills shiver up and down the spine. The doctor detects no pulse or respiration. The hand he touches is cold and nonresponsive. The doctor certifies to the death. Some time later, the eyelids begin to flutter, consciousness returns, and the certifiably deceased person awakens - only to find him or herself in a sealed coffin. This horrendous vision of being "buried alive" was common in the nineteenth and early twentieth centuries (Mackay, 1880). Although the number of such instances was almost certainly exaggerated, it is also almost certain that live burials did occur. It is the fantasy and fear, however, that most concerns us here. What is the most unthinkable, unacceptable way to die? For some people, it was the thought of being alive in death, of urgently but vainly attempting to break though the shackles of a mistaken death that is now destined to become authentic.

So much for the history of catastrophic dying, or for as much of it as we can deal with here. It is time now to touch upon the realities and fantasies with which hospice must contend today and tomorrow.

The Hospice and "Safe Death"

As you well know, it is one or another type of cancer that has most often produced the life-threatening situation that leads to hospice care. In the National Hospice Demonstration Study, for example, more than 90% of the patients had cancer-related diagnoses. Although most hospice organizations have offered their services to people with a variety of illnesses, it is not too far off the mark to observe that in its formative years, the hospice movement has served largely as a humane and competent response to lives threatened by cancer. Through its work, hospice has exercised an educational influence over both health care providers and the public, an influence that appears still to be on the rise. Several of these influences seem especially relevant to our conference.

First, it appears that the interaction between cancer and hospice care has given society a general model for the dying process. The famous (or infamous) five stages described by Kubler-Ross (1969) require what Glaser and Strauss (1968) years ago classified as a "lingering trajectory", in other words, the considerable length of time that people continue to live with some fatal illnesses. That the Kubler-Ross stage theory has serious flaws and limitations is not the point here. What is the point is that a strong tendency has developed to consider all dying within a framework that is appropriate for many people who are afflicted with cancer, but which is not appropriate for people with a variety of other afflictions that will claim their lives.

Next, we may observe that some of the excessive anxieties associated both with cancer and with the dying process have been alleviated to some extent through hospice work and through so-called "death education". Compared with, say twenty years ago, more people feel that a cancer diagnosis is not necessarily a death sentence, and more also feel that they will be spared agony and despair even when the end does grow near. Less often does "cancer" automatically translate into "dying", and less often does "dying" translate into absolute panic. In my own experience, at least, I find that many people see the last phase of life as having something of its own pattern and style - a new, formidable, threatening and unique phase of life to be sure, but one through which they might be able to pass with a certain measure of security. In other words: hospice has helped to encourage the hope of a "safe death". One may escape the worst of indignities; one may escape unremitting and unbearable pain; one may instead remain mentally and emotionally in touch with self and world and enjoy the support of sensitive and competent people. The hospice-assisted passage through life to death is "safe" in its protection from the catastrophic visions we have already reviewed, and it is "safe" because the individual's own basic values and sense of identity are confirmed rather than assaulted. This, I admit, is an idealized version, but it is not without some basis in reality. Most important for our purposes here is the expectation: I can live safely within my innermost ideas, feelings and intimate relationships while I live at all.

The situation I have just offered for your consideration can rightly be regarded as an improvement, an encouraging development. However, there is danger in the over-reliance on terminal cancer as the general model for dying, and danger in the related assumption that we now really do have a more mature understanding of death. Please bear with me for just another few minutes so that we may at least start to explore some of the emerging challenges to the success already achieved by hospice.

The first two challenges deserve more attention than we can give them here because they have rapidly been overtaken by an even more powerful menace. The possibility of being kept alive in a helpless, vegetative condition has become a major, even a dominant fear for some people. I hear it often from elderly men and women, but it is not limited to any one particular age group. Behind their reality-based concerns one can also hear resonances from the forgotten - or has it been forgotten? - fear of live burial. The prospect of being, in effect, alive and dead at the same time, is felt as so catastrophic by some people that they contemplate and may actually commit suicide. This prospect has also led to a great deal of legislative activity to provide the option for discontinuing a subhuman form of existence. Vegetative life, then, is a form of dying that for many people takes the shape of degrading rather than safe death.

Alzheimer's disease and dementias of this general type have also become of increased concern to both professional caregivers and the public, at least in the United States. The anxieties are expressed most often by those who live and work with Alzheimer victims, and by relatives who fear that this fate might befall them as well. It is not unusual for the spouse or child of an Alzheimer victim to express their own sense of being tortured. How painful and unnatural it is to see the face and frame of a person they have loved for so many years, but to come up against a mind that has gone blank. This variant form of death-in-life provides the stuff of nightmares for some people and has also provoked suicidal thoughts.

Whether horizontal, as in a vegetative state, or vertical, as in the empty shell of a brain-damaged Alzheimer victim, these images refuse to conform to the vision of "safe death". The anguish created by such unacceptable forms of dying has only occasionally come to the door of hospice. The third and final challenge, however, is one that threatens to knock on any if not every door.

Acquired Immune Deficiency Syndrome has rapidly become a new threat on both the reality and the fantasy level. Unfortunately, it has proven difficult not only to treat and prevent AIDS, but also to help the public distinguish between reality and fantasy. Even hospice with its proven record of accomplishment is for now at a disadvantage. The formidable bio-medical problems that AIDS presents are enveloped by an equally formidable atmos- phere of tension and dread. May I propose that the growing intensity of this reaction also owes much to fantasies that are starting to break free of their psychological constraints. AIDS has most of the elements that are necessary for a thoroughly catastrophic vision of death. The death-in-life appearance of the body that marked advanced tuberculosis is present also in AIDS. Furthermore, confusion and dementia often befall the AIDS victim in the later stages of the disease. The death of breath and the death of mind are intensified by the death-through-sex connection. The association here is even more unacceptable to the general public than was the case with syphilis - and syphilis was itself stigma enough. Because AIDS has become linked in particular with homosexuality, the stigma is exceptionally fierce. In the public's heart there is much less inclination to forgive the person who may have contracted his death through " unnatural" intercourse. Further- more, there is also the view that AIDS is the product of a "dirty" life, and of a tainted spirit who dared to flaunt God's moral laws. Fear and revulsion are further magnified by the fact that AIDS often claims people in the prime of their lives - it is no unobtrusive scavenger that carries off those who society has already half-forgotten.

At least one more turn of the screw must be acknowledged. AIDS is a disease that is communicated through the exchange of bodily fluids, including blood. From ancient to recent times there has been the widespread belief that "blood is the life", and we have already touched upon some of the psychological dynamics that might lie at the root of the vampire legend. AIDS has a way of speaking directly to powerful fantasies that usually remain under firm control and constraint. AIDS is the "unsafe" death par excellence. AIDS is the disease that does not attract sympathy. AIDS is the disease that does not abide by the rules established for the general model of dying inspired through hospice care of cancer patients.

AIDS is the death toward which our unconscious fantasies surge. It is the death in which a diabolic anti-self, a perverted angel, turns upon the victim with many of the terrors history has witnessed or invented. It is the death that appears among the most dangerous because it is among the most encompassing - the victim's entire life may be stigmatized and destroyed: the past as well as the future.

In the United States we are currently exposed to a mass media campaign for "safe sex". There is obviously a good deal of merit to this idea. However, it is also an exercise in self-deception to believe that sex - or love - can be "safe". What person of experience and sensitivity believes one can venture without risk? It may also be an exercise in self-deception to believe that hospice or any other human agency can provide for "safe death".

Nevertheless, the same sensitivity and determination that has been brought to hospice's current achievements might also be directed to the menace of a disease that not only destroys life but that subjects the victim to the most horrendous assaults from a public opinion that is driven in part by its own inflamed fantasies. Just recently a family home was destroyed by a firebomb. Why? Because the children in the family were carriers of the AIDS virus and other parents did not want them to attend the local school. This firebomb was, I believe, a blast from Hell - from the Hell of nightmare fantasies. My own bias, as a psychologist, is that we begin this difficult educational and sensitization process right where we ourselves live - in our own hearts and minds. Perhaps then, we will be in a position to offer something useful to others. Whatever course we take, however, hospice cannot for long ignore the anxieties re-awakened by AIDS, nor endorse the fantasy of a "safe death" for everybody.

We might also want to challenge the assumption that old people live but to die, and that their final days are not frought with peril simply because we prefer to believe that dying is as natural to the aged as living is to the young.

REFERENCES

Aries, P., 1981, "The Hour of our Death", Alfred A. Knopf, New York.
Glaser, B.G. and Strauss, A.L., 1968, "Time for Dying", Aldine, Chicago.
Kastenbaum, R., 1979, Healthy dying: a paradoxical quest continues,
    Journal of Social Issues, 35: 185-206.
Kubler-Ross, E., 1969, "On Death and Dying", Macmillan, New York.
Mackay, G.E., 1880, Premature burials, Popular Science Monthly, 16:389-397.
Mor, V., Greer, D. and Kastenbaum, R., (in press), "The Hospice Experiment:
    Is it Working?", John Hopkins University Press, Baltimore.
Twigg, G., 1984, "The Black Death: A Biological Appraisal", Batsford, London.
Yeomans, P.A., 1986, The vampire as a psychological metaphor, Unpublished
    Thesis, Antioch (Ohio) University.

THE INNER WEB

Michael Murphy

Albany Medical College
Albany, N.Y., USA

Jorge Luis Borges wrote a powerful tale of a man who dreamed up a son.
Later, when he himself was dying, he discovered that he, too, was an illusion
having been the dream of someone else's imagination. Borges was not
referring to the dreams that occur during normal sleep which seem to be
manifestations of our attempt to integrate our inner and outer worlds. He
recognized that so many of us seem to be awake, but live our waking lives
as if we are asleep and dreaming, and his story was about this illusion of
wakefulness.

We dream up and have dreams for our children, and even in the giving of
a name enmesh them in the memories and fantasies of someone else. Perhaps
we name them after a favored relative or simply add a Roman numeral to our
own name. Little wonder that they sometimes believe that they have failed
or have been a disappointment in never quite fulfilling the dreams of their
parents! Children, too, dream up their parents, investing them with powers
and attributes which are knitted and woven from their imagination and may
have little in common with their reality as people. Imagination and the
ability to dream are uniquely human characteristics, and the stimuli come
both from the outside world through the senses, particularly the visual, and
from some kind of inner soul-sense or insight which appears to be beyond
our usual physical perception. Imagination and dreaming may be inspiring
and creative gifts which help us to expand our viewpoints of both self and
others, but they can also be fascinating digressions to knowing and being
awake. Getting to know ourselves and others requires that we allow
unfiltered and unjudged perceptions to penetrate us rather than make
assumptions and imagine or dream that somehow, magically, we know them.

This paper is about waking up to ourselves and those we care about before
it is too late, for we need to be fully awake before we can say 'hello',
and saying hello is a necessary prelude to saying goodbye.

How do we get to know a person? With young children it is easy. There
is neither mask nor artiface. In a loving environment they make known their
needs, hold no resentments, quickly let go of hurt, smile hello and wail
goodbye. Their inner person is accessible and available because it is simply
surrounded by a soft and permeable membrane like that of an emerging egg.
Very quickly, however, the shell becomes hard and we seem to become more
preoccupied with its fabrication than with experiencing and developing the
soul within.

The shell has been described in terms of defense mechanisms or personality or character armor. We cover it with a whole array of costumes, adopt poses, play roles and fill our stage with goods and chatels in order to become disguised from ourselves and others. When dying, the games, goods and costumes are all of no avail. The shell becomes very fragile and may even break down. How odd that we are so afraid of "breaking down" when breaking down the elaborate barricades we have erected offers the only entrance into the soul where we can say "hello"! So breaking down is the prelude, and suffering is the process by which the shell is penetrated, and we need great courage and support to break this steely barrier that we have spent our whole lives in constructing.

What lies within the shell? Jung spoke of our shadow side; the side of ourselves that we have great difficulty in acknowledging, and from which emanates our rage, destructiveness, and the knowledge of our own death. It is difficult to accept because, like our bodily shadow, it is not readily visible so that we are unaware of it most of the time, and may even deny its very existence. But it is there and a part of us, and acceptance or gently passing through this shadow side is necessary for completeness and for connection. It is as if, deep within, lies the seed of our rebirth which will only germinate if we pass through the shadow and touch it. The shadow will lighten if we allow permeability of the shell or if it is broken down as so often happens in far-advanced illness. There are two important and related forces which assist this process: Firstly, the coming to the use of our senses and secondly, the discovery of our connective unconscious.

Most often, the senses are used in the service of the defensive shell. We look, photograph and store away visual pictures, but often fail to see! Insight is seeing beyond that which is simply recorded by the eyes. It is as if the eyes are part of the shell and there is another process required to allow penetration leading to some lightening or enlightenment within the soul. So it is with touch. We shake hands, but often our hands are but feelers and extensions of the shell, and we neither touch nor are touched by one another. Sometimes we listen but neither hear a word nor sense the sounds between the words. Coming to the use of our senses means that we recognize them as more than recording devices and allow ourselves to be receptive, vulnerable, and penetrated so that the soul and the imagination are constantly changed by what we see, hear, and touch in those around us. The world also offers so much, but we need to allow it to penetrate our sleepy and cynical covering if it is to soothe the shadow. We have all experienced great peace and awe at seeing some of the wonders of the earth, and yet we usually believe that we must wait for a vacation in the Rockies or by the sea in order to "relax" and allow in the renewing magic that nature provides! It is all around if we wake up and open our eyes and allow ourselves to be penetrated by the sounds and silences as well as the touch of the earth.

We are all connected to one another, and yet we spend much energy in our lives declaring our independence, magnifying our differences and exaggerating or being captivated by variations in the color and shape of our shells. The human body is a wonder-full example of connectedness and of a harmonically interrelated gathering of cells held together by a "Connective Unconscious". The cells are not competitive with one another unless they are malignant. They share information and nutrition, and it is as if they "know" how ridiculous it would be for one cell to assert its worth or superiority over another or that Right were better than Left! Interdependence is a prerequisite for both growth and survival of the whole, and independence fosters the danger of chaos and cancer.

Even collectively, we are beginning to realize our interconnectedness, and in these days of instant electronic communication are beginning to see the world as a global village with peace as an imperative if we are to survive. The vast network of information available about each individual might suggest that we are much known or at least instantly knowable. These statistics simply relate to the make-up of our personal and collective shells, and all this data does little to help us know ourselves or one another, and may serve as a distraction from our looking within to discover the connective unconscious web which binds us all and is the linkage to real knowing. This web provides intimacy to self and others in the present, and also protectively links the generations through genes and scenes and myth and history, and, after death of the shell, it provides continuity as our internal essence lives on through our linkages with others. It is the uncovering of this inner web which enables us to say hello and goodbye.

So end-stage cancer and other illnesses which remind us that we have a short time to live offer us the opportunity to detach ourselves from the numbing business of building shells and barriers and risk breaking through to the center of ourselves and others. If our shadow side is off limits, anger is taboo, admitting depression a sin and even the expression of love is only in things done rather than things said, we are locked in and will live and die alone in the shadow of lonely despair, even when surrounded by family. Looking within at our shadow, we can forgive our nastiness and face death, and in some miraculous way it becomes lighter. If we who are dying can offer this vulnerability to those who surround us, it becomes an invitation for them to do the same. This process is a revivification of our connectedness, and the web connecting us all is almost palpable and visible at such times.

In our Hospice work, we attempt to facilitate and make manifest this connectedness through family meetings which are gatherings including the person who has an advanced illness together with all those available who mean the most to him. This is a time for telling stories. The facts are of little importance because they are but the residual imprints of fossils on the shell. What matters are the melange of sensory impressions which have penetrated the shell, many happy and loving, others sad and loathsome.

So the "patient" tells the assembly the story of his illness and the fears and worries which still accompany it and the fears and worries and love which have usually remained locked within. The witnesses simply listen and try to hear. If they really hear, and allow themselves to become in touch with and touched by the knowledge of their own shadow and death as well as that of the story-teller, a real connection in the web of the connective unconscious is made. The patient continues by telling stories and myths about each of the assembled persons - some humorous, some sad, some very painful, some loving. Even the painful ones need to be told. For example, the pain inflicted by a dying parent who had been actively alcoholic in the past is often very great and usually neither acknowledged nor forgiven, by himself or by others. Telling the story from all sides, accompanied by recollections of the felt, seen and heard pain allows for this shadowy era to be acknowledged by each family member all together perhaps for the first time. Only then can it be forgiven and let go, and the shadow lightens a little, and more strands in the connecting web are woven together replacing the barriers. At this time we also tell the stories and myths of other deaths and losses which have never been told from inside the soul. Failure to do this compounds our sense of grief and loss so that we are not fully attentive to the individual whose life we are celebrating and to whom we need to say goodbye, and it is often quite unclear for whom the bell tolls.

In summary, saying hello is waking up from our dreams, seeing with insight, listening, hearing, and being touched by another. It is loving, it is laughing and making manifest the strands of the connective web that links us all. It is the essence of religion (re - ligio: the thing which binds) which is simply the celebration of our connectedness in the present and with both past and future. It is forgiveness of ourselves and others which in turn lightens the shadow. After that, saying goodbye is simply the touching, penetrating sadness and pain of letting go, for there is nothing more to say.

TERMINAL CARE: FROM A SOCIOLOGICAL PERSPECTIVE

Raymond Illsley

University of Bath
Bath, UK

Professionals in the field of terminal care, and in particular those working in the hospice movement are aware that they take part in an activity which departs radically from accepted past practice, which rejects and criticises the actions and standards of their professional colleagues, which introduces new concepts, new methods and which stands slightly to one side of the mainstream of conventional health care. They are also aware that their approach is itself criticised and frequently misrepresented, partly because its benefits are available only to the few, partly because it is seen as dangerously close to the controversial issue of euthanasia, on which our society has not quite made up its mind. That feeling of being at the cutting edge of thought and practice of having enemies out there but not yet within, produces a sense of pioneering, of enthusiasm and commitment.

It is my impression that these professionals are in fact well past that early pioneering stage, in the UK at least, and are already beginning to capitalise on demonstrated successes. Indeed it may be opportune henceforth to bear in mind what will happen when the hospice movement becomes a well-accepted or even a routine, service.

Some of these perspectives were too qualitative, theological and generally a-scientific to have meaning for me and I cannot comment upon them. I do, however, understand and appreciate the point that death itself has no intrinsic meaning but only the meaning given to it by the perceiver. This is described as an existentialist perspective. I would regard it as good sound conventional sociology and it is highly relevant to the perceptions and images of death and dying of other cultures and other historical periods. We forget too easily how far and how fast we have come in recent decades and on what different realities our forefathers' perceptions, and perspectives were based.

For other research purposes I went back recently to look at the death rates of 1921 in Britain - two years after I was born. I was reminded that, at that time, 27% of deaths occurred before the age of 15, that 42% occurred between 16 and 64 and that only 35% died at 65 or later. In other words, child death and death in the prime of adult life were each almost as common as death of the elderly. And yet by 1921 we had already begun to bring down the rates of early death massively from their 19th century levels. The whole experience of death in our society has changed. The turnover of birth and death was faster and greater and the sight of a hearse and the knowledge

of a child death, of a young parent, was not an uncommon experience. Child
death today has become and has been mentioned several times in this meeting
as the tragic, deplored, wasteful but exceptional phenomenon. Epidemio-
logists frequently use death before the age of 65 as a criteria of premature
death these days - and that has already become an out-of-date definition in
some societies with an average expectation of life at birth of 73, 76 or
even 79. Today, death is a comparatively rare experience, which hits
families infrequently and where consequently we have little personal preparation. We have yet to adjust to that situation, as we have to prolonged
terminal illness, and to develop new and appropriate practices, rituals and
meanings. If Victorian or earlier perspectives seem unreal to us, we should
remember that they were perspectives in a quite different reality.

Reference is frequently made to the isolating experience of death, and
to the fear of closeness and contact. Dr Richardson, in describing her quite
fascinating research on 'nest eggs' stored by old people, reminded us of how
close we were to the workhouse and death 'on the parish'. This makes it
easier to recall that most of these deaths, like most deaths at the time,
came from infectious diseases, the scourge of our 19th century cities. It
was in the mid-19th century that research first conclusively showed how the
great lethal infections came about through proximity to or contact with
infected persons. Fear of contact with dying people had a powerful and
logical rationale. For many people illness, but above all lethal illness,
contained many elements of the fearful unknown.

We should also be careful about making comparisons, good or bad, with
developing societies of today or agrarian societies of the past. It is too
east to abstract what was good and forget what was and is bad. They were
and are very different from each other as well as from us. The buildings
(Pyramids, temples and churches) the few written records or remembered folk-
tales, the religions, all tell a story, but they are difficult to interpret
realistically and the story was often understood and lived by a tiny elite
whose lives and deaths mattered and may be remembered in myths and monuments
(even the Christian saints were overwhelmingly upper class in their origins)
whilst the mass of ordinary human beings lived and died in forgotten misery.
I doubt very much whether they were aware of, let alone lived by, the noble
philosophies often attributed to them.

The hospice movement is outstandingly a creation of the late 20th
century, occurring among peoples for whom death is a relative rarity (every
70 years instead of every 25) occurring largely to elderly people, often
following a long terminal illness rather than an acute infection, and in a
society which knows much about the causes of illness. Many of the older
attitudes remain in our culture and in our services and institutions but the
dynamics of life and living in the century to come will inevitably lead to
the wider and wider acceptance of the morality and customs of the hospice
approach. That doesn't make us superior to the poor old Victorians, just
very fortunate.

Another theme pursued through reflection on terminal care has been that
of honesty, of candid open relationships with dying persons. Again, the
hospice movement has taken a great leap forward in telling dying patients
their diagnosis and prognosis, in discussing all the implications with them,
and giving them support in their final months and days. In this respect,
it is again a creature of the late 19th century. Less than 20 years ago,
my Research Unit was asked to study events, practices and relationships in
what was predominantly a ward for cancer patients. They had not been told
of the diagnosis. In practice the great majority had themselves observed
and interpreted carefully and knew; and similarly with the prognosis about
the outcome and the length of time left to them. But the mutual silence

was maintained. This does still occur but openness has broken out all over
the place and not just in hospices, and not just in relation to cancer and
terminal illness. Perhaps some of the past practice stemmed from genuine
medical uncertainties about diagnosis and outcome and the doctor's reluctance
to be seen to be wrong. Some stemmed from medical, and particularly surgical
arrogance to 'patients'. And this was the more easy to maintain in the
presence of lay ignorance and deference. Greater openness is evident in all
fields of medicine and illness under the impact of social and educational
change. It still, outside the hospice movement, has farthest yet to go in
relation to terminal illness and the elderly.

And what of the future? Professionals, I think, face that future from
a base of, admittedly brief, but nevertheless solid achievement - in terms
of human being treated, supported and comforted, of sharp challenges to
earlier attitudes and practice, and of an impact upon attitude and practice
in more conventional settings outside the hospice movement. The medical,
institutional world of death and dying will never be the same again. In this
sense, your patient has been not only the terminally ill patient, or even
their friends and relatives, but a wider society which cannot ignore a more
understanding and humane approach.

There is a long way to go. There is scepticism among people who know
little, about what can be and is being done. To dispel that requires time,
but also publicity. There is also hostility among those who ought to know
better - partly because it challenges old ideas and their own practice,
partly because resource constraints prevent the approach from being extended
across all institutions and centre and because, in consequence, the tiny
proportion of hospice patients are seen as a privileged minority. Clearly
the ultimate goal must be the incorporation of the hospice philosophy into
the whole health service. This is a formidable goal for the future requiring
public and professional and political re-education.

Research was mentioned a necessary component of re-education programmes.
A start has been made, much of it still within orthodox settings. The continued interest of Ann Cartwright in this field is itself a comfort. She
demonstrates by her scientific rigour, the standards of scientific research
required to convince a sceptical audience - just as she also demonstrated
at this meeting the immense methodological and conceptual difficulties yet
to be faced. Other research is rising up within the hospice movement itself
and some good examples were evident in the presentations at this meeting.
There will be pressure from conventional funding bodies for research to
conform to certain research conventions which draw heavily on research in
the physical sciences. I think particularly of randomised controlled trials.
They are very useful - in moderation and in their proper place. There are
very few questions in research on health services or on human and social
experiences which are suitable or adaptable for such conventional research.
What is required is a range of quantitative, qualitative, documentary,
observational, anthropological, historical, etc, etc research. It all needs
to conform to the criteria that it should attempt rigorously to falsify its
own conclusions. New movements sometimes like to think that that are per-
secuted by research funding bodies, and they sometimes are. Some of the
stuffier bodies will say that they are sympathetic, have looked around for
good applications, but none of them meet their scientific criteria. The
first social science application on Aids, made two years before the public
panic, was turned down on these grounds by every research council and
funding body in sight. Today they fight to accept it. My own judgment is
that research on terminal illness and on hospice approaches is already
acceptable and what is needed is the attraction of first class research
workers into the field.

THE PROBLEMS OF DEATH AND DYING FROM A PSYCHOANALYTIC PERSPECTIVE

Renée Sebag-Lanoë

Paul Brousse Hospital
Villejuif, France

In 1977, I was assigned as a doctor to a geriatric unit specialising
in chronic care hospitalization which was located in the near Paris suburbs.
The patients I was responsible for were very elderly people. They were on
the average over 80 years old. I also knew that sooner or later they would
all die in our midst. As well as being preoccupied with improving the
quality of medical treatment given to them, I also wanted to improve the
quality of life within the institution, and to improve the conditions of
death for these very elderly people. I was familiar with Elizabeth Kubler-
Ross's (1969) work on the psychology of dying people. I knew that in
England there was a hospice where the doctors were successfully using morphine to treat the suffering of terminal cancer patients. But we were in
France: and this work was only known to a very few individuals. The notions
of accompanying dying patients, and of palliative treatment were still not
in medical vocabulary. Nonetheless, a book written by the famous oncologist,
Léon Schwartzenberg and the journalist, Louis Viansson-Ponte, entitled
"Changer la mort" (Changing Death) was published in 1977. This beautiful,
moving book, which foresaw active euthanasia negotiated between doctor and
terminal patient, was incontestably to mark French medical and social thinking on the subject, and was to influence doctors' behaviour.

What attitude was I supposed to take towards the dying patient? Was I
to desert him as I had all too often seen happen in many hospital units?
I didn't feel that I had the right to. Was I to desperately go on trying
to save him right up to the end? This denial of death seemed all the more
absurd to me as the patients I was treating were very old and their death
was in fact something completely natural. Was I artificially to precipitate
inescapable death with some medicinal injection? This "clean" solution
didn't satisfy me either. It wasn't a question of a religious attitude,
but rather, I couldn't recognize my role as a doctor in it; nor the reasons
why I had chosen this profession. Those were my internal conflicts. I was
looking for my way. I was looking for a model of death which was appropriate
for the old people who were entrusted to our care; appropriate for their
families and for ourselves, the care deliverers who were to live with them
for months and even years.

Since my arrival, I had undertaken to work very closely with the nurses
and orderlies. I knew that I would be able to do nothing by myself alone,
and that their role with the elderly patients was really primordial. As a
result, we met frequently to communicate, and to discuss all the daily

material problems. And there were many of them, for at that time our means were still very limited in this sector which was under-developed, under-medicalized, and very little appreciated in French hospitals. Accordingly, in the course of one of these meetings we tried to deal with the problem of dying patients with the help of a psychologist and a physiotherapist who were particularly sensitive to it. I was in fact convinced that we could only change things together and only after talking about them. But we were still denying the existence of one problem : for care deliverers patients were never actually dying. They were only very, very tired! It was barely possible to talk about death. Our defenses were too strong. We were still living with the modern taboo about death which various French historians and sociologists had exposed very well. What were we to do? I was lucky enough to have the psychoanalyst, Hugues Liborel for a friend, and I spoke to him periodically about this new professional reality which I had been discovering for several months. Was he the one who had suggested it ; or was I? He was to come once a month to help me, and the care deliverers who wanted to, to think about our situation.

This was the spring of 1979. The beginnings were difficult. Very quickly the group found itself rejected by the unit. What was a psycho-analyst doing in a chronic care unit? Someone who didn't see patients, and who kept his hands clean! So for one year we met once a month in Hugues Liborel's own home. There he received a small group of six or seven motivated people, determined to go into these issues in depth. In the re-assuring warmth of the group, we dealt with our identity as a team confronted with our patients' death, and with our own anxiety about death. We would even imagine our own needs and expectations in the same situation. This self analysis was to allow us to truly begin to look at and to listen to our dying patients and to try to meet their needs. For us, it was an indispensible and fundamental stage. In fact, if anxiety which inherently has the characteristics of indecision and absence of any real object is not recog-nized and expressed by staff first, it can easily take the patient himself for its object, and thus prevent or at least interfere greatly with any relationship with the patient (1987). Later on we were to meet in the unit once a month. The group was always to remain limited in number and multi-disciplinary, comprising six to ten people who were motivated by different technical specializations and levels of hierarchy, doctors, nurses, super-visors, physiotherapists and social workers, and the like. From one session to the next and from one month to the next, we spoke together about our dying patients and our problems. Every process of dying is different, and every dying person teaches us something new. One noteworthy fact : the majority of care deliverers in the unit didn't participate in these meetings with the psychoanalyst. Nonetheless new styles of behaviour spread throughout the institution at a disconcerting speed. This we will come back to. Some years later, in 1985, we were able to conceptualize our objectives. Our aims were simple :

1. To avoid moving or isolating the terminal patient, in order to spare him the trauma which - at the very moment when physical comfort and serenity are primordial - a change in material and relational surroundings always entails.

2. To treat physical suffering every time it occurs, using analgesics, notably morphine administered every 4 hours, just as we learned from the the head pharmacist in our hospital - who knew St. Christopher's potion - and as we learned later from Dr Therese Vanier whom we went to see in London, and also from Doctor Michele Salamagne who did much to spread these techniques in France, and who translated Saunders and Baines' book, "Living with Dying : The Management of Terminal Disease" (1983) into French.

3. We also try to feed and hydrate the patient as naturally as possible while avoiding any useless tubes.

4. We seek to realize his comfort particularly emphasizing nursing which is of course very important with very old patients who are nearly always bed-ridden in the terminal phase.

5. We also seek to favour as much as possible the presence of the family by making visiting hours more flexible so that they become open, day as well as night, and by improving the reception which families get in the institution and by giving them the help and support necessary in difficult moment.

6. We also try particularly hard to maintain communication with dying elderly people by learning as the need arises how to resort to observing gestures, mimicry and looks, and how to use hand contact, and how to bring everything which we call non-verbal into play. We do this in order to try to meet the individual needs and desires of each dying person while respecting each one's unique identity.

Very quickly, however, we realized that there is no ready-made formula for accompanying someone's dying; that it can only be an attempt which requires a constant renewal of goals ; that nothing is ever truly acquired, but always has to be done again. Accompanying - no more than desperate therapeutic search for a cure, or euthanasia - is not the solution to the problem. The analysis which we were pursuing with Hugues Liborel allowed us to escape fantasies of mastery and omnipotence which could have plagued us. In fact, we were gradually finding where our problems were and where they would always exist :

1. First there is the problem of recognizing that an old person is going to die.

If prognosis is relatively easy when an elderly person has a fatal disease beyond a certain stage of its development, like a cancer or another malignant growth, it proves to be much more difficult in many other cases. How indeed are we to know if an elderly person's acute illness is a curable episode which we will have the pleasure and duty of treating effectively, or a terminal illness? There are hardly any rules or ready-made formulas for analyzing this sort of situation. Of course, we have to take the objective clinical and biological medical situation into account, but we mustn't neglect what the patient himself says, nor his physical behaviour or his cooperation with treatment. Naturally the signs described by Hippocrates retain their value, but they are very late ones. Of course, the patient's symbolic language can throw light on his future evolution. But in order to modify our attitudes to treatment can we base ourselves with certainty on the few words about departure, returning, journeys, home-land, heaven, mothers or other loved ones who have already passed away? We must never lose sight of the fact that what an elderly patient says about death may certainly have something to do with signalling phenomena as described by Kubler-Ross (1969) and by Exton-Smith (1961), and as we have ourselves observed several times (Sebag-Lanoe, 1986), but that they may also have something to do with an authentic depressive syndrome which is perfectly curable. Some biological parameters may also have prognostic value, (Moulias et al., 1986), but here again certainty is difficult and definitely easier after the fact, that is, once the patient is deceased. In these moments of uncertainty, contact in meetings between different care deliverers proves very valuable ; here also Saunders and Baines's schema takes on its full significance. It shows us that there is no hard and fast border between palliative and terminal treatment on the one hand, and curative treatment on the other. There is instead a continuum and an evolving strategy which constantly allows us to adapt treatment and type of care to the patient's condition. Nonetheless we are constantly exposed to doubt, denial and guilt. Doubt with respect to our knowledge and understanding of these situations. Denial which may show up at any time with a particular patient or because several deaths one after the other may - at least in our imagination - put our competence into question. Finally, guilt : for either having done too much or not enough.

2. The second problem we have identified is hearing about death in the present tense ; that is, hearing the patient talk about his own death.

Our training never prepared us for that ; training which takes place in a society which as Aries, (1975) states "has decided once and for all that death is no longer any of its business". How then can we not help running away from the problem and why mustn't we run away from it? There is hardly any other solution than first talking together about our fears, about the trouble we have listening, and about our own anxiety. An elderly person's death is certainly more acceptable for people in medical professions than the death of a child or of a young adult. It still upsets us though because it brings us face to face with the inevitability of death and with our own mortality. This condition - being mortal - is a rather abstract notion which is always difficult to accept - especially when one is young, and especially when one belongs to a society which no longer encourages its discovery. Here there is real work to be done, a sort of re-education, so that first of all we can get rid of this anxiety. In this opened up space we can re-discover our eyes and ears for others. This openness and accessibility constantly have to be rebuilt, for nothing is ever truly acquired. Do our elderly patients talk to us about death? And how do they do it? Direct explicit references to it are actually relatively rare ; because our elderly patients generally say little in their last days. What is essential is said symbolically so that one may or may not hear it and interpret it. Above all, it is communicated non-verbally : through looks, signs, and gestures which are heavy with meaning for the person who is able and wants to perceive them. When the message is clear, for example "I feel that I'm dying", it's much more a question of being open to, and recognizing an experience with respect and understanding than one of answering a question with a yes or a no. Indeed only silence seems appropriate in these moments, for the elderly person often already knows much more than we do about what's happening and what's going to happen to him. We can therefore risk the question: "Why do you say that?" "Do you feel something in particular?" It is a way of showing the patient that we have been listening to him. This effort over our anxiety and towards accessibility we have to make over and over again. It is a way of staying ready to see and to hear the other person while avoiding giving him what Mount (1978) calls "reflected fear", that is, that fear which the patient sees in the eyes of those around him. In geriatrics it is all the more necessary as there is often an enormous gulf between the person giving the treatment and the person receiving it : the person giving the treatment, generally young, has his young person's anxieties about death, whereas the elderly person - as long as he doesn't suffer too much and we don't disturb him - views his approaching death with relative serenity. As Kubler-Ross, (1969), writes : "One type of patient will arrive at acceptance without any help or with very little help from those around him other than silent understanding which abstains from interferance. This is the rather elderly patient who feels that he is at the end of his life, and who has worked and suffered, raised children, and accomplished his purpose in life. This type of patient will have discovered the meaning of life and looking back on his active years, feels a certain contentment". Many studies in the literature on this subject emphasize the relative serenity of elderly people towards death, and all our personal and collective experience in this domain corroborates this notion.

3, The third problem is that of accompanying a dying person's body.

A dying person's body is still, of course, a living one, but passing from the world of the living to that of the dead it is becoming a corpse. Can't this dying person pull me along, take me along with him on his inexorable journey towards death, to the land of the dead? This is the ancestral fear of being pulled along by the dying person, and these fears are abundantly illustrated by folklore, as the psychoanalyst, Michel de M'Uzan, (1977) explains. This fear is inside us, in our body. It is like the fear of being contaminated : Won't this living body, which is already carrying death in it, pass it on to me? All the more so because the other person's present situation sends me back intensely to my own weakness, and the precariousness of my own body. The relation between the person giving the treatment and the person receiving it is not only a relationship of words, it is also, and perhaps primarily, especially in terminal situations, a body to body relationship between the body of the care deliverer and that of the care receiver. Here again, there is distance to maintain and constantly rebuild between my body and that of the dying person. This distance allows for a true relationship, even a tactile one, and good bodily treatment. Here again, there is anxiety which has to be discarded beforehand; a heavy burden which we have to take apart at least partly before we can take charge of the body of the person who is dying. But this dying body also makes me suffer in my own body. Even when the patient is comforted, when he isn't suffering anymore, when he isn't complaining, there is still this body which is being irremediably transformed under my very eyes : there are still these wounds and these decubiti which distress me every day. So, how am I to comfort my patient properly : how am I to give him or her my hand, to touch and bandage this body, and put all my technical effectiveness in the service of the person who is dying, if I cannot first recognize, name, and express my own suffering that I feel, me, the person who is looking at him and touching him? This task is all the more important for us in that this body to body relationship can become the essential part of our communicating, which has now become mute. Because the elderly person is aphasic; or demented ; or quite simply silent. Words leave off, whereas hands keep on speaking. Here there is something absolutely essential to give and to receive. Michel De M'Uzan (1977), writes : "I am afraid that we never measure the importance of this basic contact enough ; be it limited to one hand holding another when verbal exchange has become impossible. Here there is something comparable to the single organism that the mother and the new born child make up. But beyond anxiety and suffering there is still our inaptitude in communicating without words. We haven't learned ; we aren't used to it. We don't know reality very well and we often underestimate it; it and the power and meaning of non-verbal communication. Here there is a need to learn and a chance to discover.

4. The fourth problem is that of interpreting requests to die.

What indeed does a patient's request to die correspond to? To a request, to a wish, or to the will to die? asks the anthropologist, Louis-Vincent Thomas (1985). Is it a real request or a cry of suffering or despair from an individual in distress, or a call for help? And who is being requested? The person who has the authority to prescribe lethal drugs ; or other people, that is, those who administer the medicine? There is sometimes a double language which we have to bring out in the open. Ambivalence is part of life ; why wouldn't the dying person be ambivalent? How are we to interpret this message and how are we to answer it? Must we take the patient at his word? Or, on the contrary, translate and convert the request into a call for help? Help not to suffer ; help not to live through this moment alone; help to stay alive right to the end. Here again we have to work. Will we only hear the death wish of the patient himself, or will we hear, at the same time and without making a distinction from the time before, that more or less conscious death wish which is connected to our own suffering which, on top of everything else, the death wish of the family, suffering also, can be added? All these untold sufferings add up. Precipitating the patient's death is not the solution. We'd better find something else. Something else for the patient, whose suffering can be relieved otherwise ; for the family whom we should also teach how to treat suffering ; and for ourselves if we want to avoid having recourse to euthanasia. To tell the truth we have only exceptionally been confronted with requests for euthanasia from elderly people. Perhaps it's because our patients are very old? Ward (1980), has shown that the acceptance of death and that of euthanasia are two very distinct things and that if acceptance of the former increases with age, that of the latter, on the other hand, diminishes. Perhaps it's also because since the beginning of our research we have been preoccupied with relieving our patients' pain, and offering understanding listening to the families? In this, we have been greatly inspired by the experience of the English hospices. And this school of thought has been fundamental to us given the existence in France of a current of thought in favour of euthanasia which was becoming commonplace in hospitals as Verspieren (1984), has pointed out clearly.

5. Finally the fifth problem is that of mourning for our patients.

We cannot of course pretend to invest ourselves in a patient and to accompany him in his last journey without paying a certain emotional price when he passes on. There is mourning to live through, and mourning to express with others. With the family, with the other elderly people, with everyone who knew and accompanied him. There is a ritual for survivors to perform which must be rediscovered and reinvented in the institution. A few words will always evoke the passing on of he or she whose name we repeat, in a staff meeting, or more informally. The care deliverers will often go to the funeral, accompanying the family in their mourning ; the other elderly people will be able if they so desire to come along for a final farewell. The deceased's bed will stay empty several days before receiving a new patient. There is a ritual of mourning which has to be reinstated so that we may better live through these successive deaths ; mourning to do and to say so that we can reinvest ourselves in new patients afterwards. This reinvention of mourning had to be done, all the more so because we staff members of a geriatric unit mix with our elderly patients for months if not years before we see them pass on. Mourning is the price to pay for true relations and true relationships. But who will say that closeness, true communication, authentic human contact – be it even at the price of tears – do not offer infinitely more susbstance to care deliverers than distance, absence of communication, or even the desertion and the guilt which accompany them?

This analysis carried out under the guidance of psychoanalyst, Hugues Liborel, has allowed us to re-establish the discussion of death in the institution, and to promote new styles of behaviour among staff members. This time and room for discussion still survive today ; as a moment for thought, for deepening and questioning practice ; as a place for analyzing institutional expression, problems and conflicts. In Hugues Liborel's opinion, the work which we have been pursuing for several years now was to allow every one of us to discern – for himself and in the group – his own way of treatment through analyzing roles and functions in a geriatric unit. Without any doubt, this had repercussions throughout the general ambience of the institution, in relations between different levels of caretakers amongst themselves, and contributed towards reducing stress in conformity with Vachon's (1987) theses. Treatment for terminal patient today makes up an integral part of our geriatric practice – in a spirit of continuity of treatment. For all that, we haven't become "specialists" in dealing with terminal patients. Our monthly average of deaths varies from 3 to 5

depending on the year, out of a population of 200 beds of octogenarians!
On the other hand, this work has, without a doubt, had repercussions in our
whole approach to the elderly patient by facilitating, notably, the handling
of all the partial deaths which major handicap and particularly dementia
represent. This experience is not unique in France for in other teams and
in particularly in cancerology units, as Goldenberg (1984) records, psychoanalysts have encouraged analysis of the the same type, and the development
of palliative treatment; and this even before an actual unit of palliative
care was opened in Paris in June 1987. A certain number of features
particular to our experiences are nonetheless worth emphasizing.

1 - From a sociological point of view : our unit like all geriatric units
     in France was and alas is still often characterized as a mouroir, a
     place to put old people to die. Accordingly, for us, our work on
     humanizing the conditions of death for our patients represented a way
     of putting death back in its rightful place in the institution, and
     also a way of fighting against the negative image which society and
     the hospital world reflected back to us. Indeed, the two books which
     set out French institutional experiences in the field, that is
     "Mourir dans la Tendresse" (Dying in tenderness) by Jomain (1984),
     and "Mourir Accompange" (Dying Accompanied) Sebag-Lanoe (1986) come
     out of chronic care units....

2 - From an anthropological point of view : we have been struck by the
     speed with which the behaviour of care deliverers was modified
     although not even the majority of them participated in the psycho-
     analytic groups. Apart from the well-known institutional phenomena
     of group dynamics and group conformity which gradually fostered talk
     about the dying patients in the course of ordinary team meetings with
     no psychoanalyst present, the need to ritualize behaviour certainly
     explains this phenomenon in part. The anthropologist, Louis-Vincent
     Thomas (1985) characterizes this phenomenon as an oblation ritual among
     different death rites which allows care deliverers to handle their
     anxiety towards dying people better.

3 - From a socio-cultural point of view : it was probably easier to re-
     discover the behaviour patterns towards dying people and death of
     French villages in the heart of 40 bed therapeutic communities - which
     we were trying to get to come alive with conviviality on the village
     model - with old people and care deliverers who due to their shared
     rural origins still remembered ancestral communal behaviour....

4 - Finally, from an analytic point of view : as we were able to discern
     with Liborel, care deliverers in geriatrics - often involved in long
     term relations with their patients - are lead to take on the role of
     a substitute family in the context of a triangular relationship with
     the elderly person and his original family. Active euthanasia would
     therefore no doubt take them back to fantasies of murdering their own
     grandparents and ancestors. This leads them to propose other types
     of behaviour. Salimpour (1986) supplies a supporting argument in this
     respect in his work, "Euthanasia. Who for? What for?" carried out
     among care deliverers in the South of France. When he asks the
     question, "in what circumstances could you envisage euthanasia?",
     extreme old age actually obtains the fewest yesses and the most nos!
     In fact, the concepts of accompanying dying people, and palliative
     treatment are doing well in French gerontological circles. As for
     psychoanalysis and the psychoanalyst himself, which were taken out of
     their normal context of operation and put in the position of collabor-
     ating with geriatrics, they had to find a way of becoming part of the
     team, and adopting a psychoanalytico-pedagogic position. The in-
     creasing recognition of the whole team's work, concretized by publicly

taking position, publishing a journal since 1982, and organizing seminars of analysis on relations with and treatment for elderly dying people since 1986, is certainly the most tangible result.

To our way of thinking, all this clearly illustrates:

- That beyond the religious aspect, treatment for dying people, and mourning represent anthropological needs which allow survivors to live better in all societies ... including the micro-societies that hospitals are.

- That they must necessarily be adapted to medical and social change, and in particular to the veritable mutation that the migration of death from the home to the hospital over the last twenty years represents.

- But that they must also be based in the socio-cultural history of the country.

- That finally, the light of analysis definitely allows care deliverers to conceptualize what they do and why they do it while at the same time, in return, enriching the psychoanalyst's thinking on old age and death.

REFERENCES

Aries, P., 1975, "Essais sur l'Histoire de la Mort en Occident", Editions du Sevil, Paris.
De M'Uzan, M., 1977, "Le Travail du Trepas in De l'art à la mort", Editions Gallimard, Paris.
Exton-Smith, A.N., 1961, Terminal illness in the aged, Lancet, 2:305-308
Goldenberg, E., 1984, Comment se forment les formateurs? Formation réciproque de l'analyste et de l'équipe soignante au sein d'un groupe des soignants, Psychologie Médicale, 16:2227-2228.
Jomain, C., 1984, "Mourir dans la Tendresse", Editions Le Ceinturion, Paris.
Kubler-Ross, E., 1969, "On Death and Dying", Macmillan, New York.
Liborel, H., 1987, Le psychanalyste et l'angoisse les soignants en geriatrie, Accompagner Bulletin, 13, Hôpital Paul Brousse, Villejuif.
Moulias, R., Proust, J., Rosenzweig, J., Nafziger, J., Debouzy, C., Wisniak, J., Congy, F., Wang, A., and Lesourd, B., 1986, Lymphopenie et infection bactériennes du signe pronostique majeur en gériatrie, La Revue de Gériatrie, 11:142-145.
Mount, B., 1978, Soins palliatifs dans les maladies terminales, Médicine de l'homme, 105:6-13.
Salimpour, A., 1986, L'Euthanasie. Pour qui? Pourquoi?, Association "Psychologie et Cancer", 4:6-15.
Saunders, C., and Baines, M., 1983, "Living with Dying: The Management of Terminal Disease", Oxford University Press, London.
Schwartzenberg, L., and Viansson-Ponte, P., 1977, "Changer la Mort", Editions Albin Michel, Paris.
Sebag-Lanoë, R., 1986 "Mourir Accompagné", Editions Desclee de Brouwer, Paris.
Thomas, L. V., 1985, "Rites de Mort", Editions Fayard, Paris.
Vachon, M., 1987, "Occupational Stress in the Care of the Critically Ill, the Dying and the Bereaved", Hemisphere Publishing Corporation, Washington.
Verspieren, P., 1984, Sur la pente de l'Euthanasie, Etudes, janvier, 4:43-54.
Ward, R., 1980, Age and Acceptance of Euthanasia, Journal of Gerontology, 35:421-431.

THE ANXIETY OF THE UNKNOWN - DYING IN A PSYCHO-EXISTENTIAL PERSPECTIVE

Jorn Beckmann and Henrik Olesen

Odense University Hospital
Odense, Denmark

THE PARABLE OF THE MUSTARD SEED

A Buddhist legend records the story of a mother who, in deep despair over her son's death, approaches Buddha for a 'cure' for her child.

Buddha explains to her that what she is looking for can be found in a few mustard seeds, but she must be certain they come from a household where death has never been.

After a while she realises that death is a cornerstone in the foundation of life. It can't be avoided through self-deception and false hopes. Afterwards, this realisation allows her to go to the funeral of her son in peace and harmony and surrender him to the flames.

This buddhist legend tells the existential story of the eternal reluctance of mankind to accept the fact of death. Ever since man has gained self-awareness and learned to reflect on himself and his condition beyond its given present, the question of the end of life has insinuated itself as an indisputable component in our anxiety.

All cultures have tried hard to reconcile themselves through their religions and philosophies.

In The Vedas - the 3000 year old religious writings of the East, the writings of Socrates and Plato up to those in our present culture and philosophy, man's basic problem has been to accept life in the light of death. According to the culture-philosopher Oswald Spengeler (1923) preoccupation with death is simply the most important element in the development of human consciousness.

In his own words:

"Man is the only creature who knows death ... at the decisive point in life, when man first becomes human and learns of his enormous loneliness in the universe, universal fear is revealed to be a purely human anxiety about death. Here is the source of the greatest spring, which first and foremost reflects thinking about death. Every religion, every branch of science, every philosophy emanates from this point".

All universal endeavours to understand death have common ground in the fact that they emanate from the primal existential anxiety which death has always awakened in man and which, unless psychologically processed, becomes a serious threat to human fellowship.

The various religious institutions and philosophical universes which have been erected everywhere are, therefore, in addition to the spiritual need which they satisfy, attempts to give death a meaningful place in our life. In certain times this has worked better than today, when the subject of death generates massive repressions in our Western culture and where the balance between individual needs and the needs of society in this borderline situation is disturbed, to the advantages of the latter.

It hasn't always been like that.

DEATH IN CULTURAL HISTORY

In the Middle Ages death was ever present. It was there physically in the form of the Plague, but it was also allowed to be admitted to consciousness.

Paintings and ornamentations demonstrated that skeletons and skulls were ever present. Increasingly naturalistic depictions of decay and half-disintegrated corpses are found in church paintings and frescos.

The great Saint of the Middle Ages, Francis of Assisi, traditionally is depicted as a figure in prayer with his hands folded around a skull, meditating on death in the hope of gaining deeper insight into life and its values.

Memento Mori - Remember death - this was the message.

This focus on the transcience of life may seem morbid today, but the reward was a hugely enhanced intensity of life. Nothing was taken for granted; focus was on what one had; attempts were made to accomplish as much as possible while time permitted - a theme which will be expanded on later.

The kind of death one would hope for today - that is, to die in one's sleep, in ignorance of the event, was, in the Middle Ages and The Renaissance, only wished upon one's enemies.

An orderly kind of death was part of an orderly life, and a number of ceremonies were an intrinsic part of dying. A will was written, psalms were chosen, and the speeches to be held were well prepared, these tasks were all in order long before death actually occurred. But the gathering of kinsmen was most important.

Friends and family would arrive to pay their respects to the dying person who, in this knowledge, was confined to bed in the all-purpose room. People stayed with the dying person during the time that remained. They said goodbye and asked for mutual forgiveness for the griefs they had caused each other.

Philippe Aries (1981) has called the attitude towards death as it was in the Middle Ages and the following centuries the "tamed death". By this he means that people were so intimate and familiar with death, that they could meet it with openness and calm.

The shift to the alienation of death in our age, began around the 18th Century when people consciously began to experience death as the absolute break with the unknown. Anxiety grew, and death became more and more difficult to accept.

A concrete example of this is seen in our reluctance to surrender our loved ones to death.

Maintenance of the grave has become accepted custom, and in the same way that the living can be visited at home, the dead can now be visited too. They are, thus, still tied to life.

Aries calls today's attitude "The forbidden death" - death is collectively repressed, suppressed, and physically banished from the home.

This orientation towards death is first and foremost directed towards the benefit of the survivors, and to the effective functioning of society.

Civilized modern man is alienated from nature in its painful aspects, and the survivors are protected from the ugliness of death and the "unproductive feelings" which result from it by the removal of the dying from the home to the hospital, where they die alone or among strangers. All endeavours is thus concentrated on minimizing fear and pain of the survivors. The prepared and tamed death of the Middle Ages has today gone "wild".

Death is also consciously banished in euphemisms such as "passed away".

Psychodynamically the growing repression tendency is a result of an increasing anxiety level. The dread which we experience in relation to death has thus become greater during the past hundred years. And at the same time, the religious and philosophical metauniverses that are culturally available for the integration of death, have lost their meaning in a world becoming increasingly pragmatic and technological.

Later on, we will look at how the collective repression of death creates serious problems in our mental balance. But first we'll look more closely at the anxiety which triggers everything.

ANXIETY OF THE UNKNOWN

People's relationship to death has been especially studied within the existentialistic tradition. And a great deal of existential philosophy is based on the specific contention, that man is the only creature than can transcend himself and his present time, to such a degree, that he can embrace his own death consciously.

Death is a key concept in existentialistic theory, because, in its essence, death condenses most of the basic characteristics of existence.

For the existentialist, existence is an unbroken chain of larger or smaller separations during which the individual is parted from the known and secure, and must venture into the unknown and the possible.

These separations arouse anxiety, partially because their inherent similarities generate the major, final separation: death - as an anxiety filled, psychological reality for the individual.

Throughout his life man is separated, or dies, in relation to specific situations, people and phases, to be born again and again into new situations, relationships and phases, from which he will also die.

The choice is for example, a daily recurring mini-separation, in which one dies in relation to some specific possibilities in order to be born into others. In this way death is constantly aroused by everyday occurrences in life, and choices and separation are just examples of some of the life conditions that make fear and death ever present.

Birth and death, which on a biological level are only experienced once, are constantly experienced at the psychological level, and one can say like St. Paul, "I die daily".

These thoughts have caused some later existential psychologists, among them Yalom (1980), to state that the anxiety of death is the basis of human life. They have demonstrated, from this perspective, how a long list of ordinary human - as well as pathological - anxiety phenomena are derived from this basic anxiety.

These analyses are consistent and reliable, but they stop one step short. In the following, the standpoint that death anxiety in itself is a derivative of an even more basic anxiety will be defended: namely the anxiety for the unknown, which also can be observed in a child before it consciously can reflect on himself and much less acknowledge or understand the reality of death!

We are here considering the empirical phenemenon which is called 7-month anxiety in developmental psychology. At this age, the child starts to react with tears and emotions when faced with a stranger, although previously he did not differentiate between the mother figure and strangers.

As soon as object consistency has been established, which according to Piaget occurs around this age, the child, now is capable of perceiving his surroundings with sufficient differentiation to distinguish the known from the unknown, reacts to the unknown with anxiety.

This pattern of behaviour is apparently universal and can be observed innumerable times in the course of development, when the individual is removed from the known and confronted with the unknown and the possible. Strangers and new situations will be met with reserve, fear, and guarded scepticism, until late in development, and for some people for the remainder of their lives. In fact, in certain primitive societies the same word is used for 'enemy' and 'stranger'.

It is likely that a state of anxiety that is almost instinctive is awakened by the unknown, and a major developmental problem arises when learning to cope with this situation appropriately.

Life begins by the individual being extruded into the unknown through violent and painful separation. This constitutes the prototype of all later experiences of anxiety, as pointed out by many psychoanalysts from Freud to Bowlby. Therefore, it seems more reasonable to talk about the separative anxiety for the unknown, as the primary basic anxiety from which anxiety for death is derived.

Anxiety for death is then only one of many manifestations of this basic anxiety. Social and individual psychological phenomena like authoritarianism, intolerance, racism, stereotyping, conformity, rigidity, and compulsiveness are all based on anxiety for the unknown and the possible. This is also true of cognitive psychological phenomena, such as intolerance of ambiguity, tendency towards premature closure, and selective perception, to name a few.

The present day growth of fear of death, along with other phenomena like authoritarianism and intolerance, is probably the result of greater anxiety of the unknown. Unemployment, the general complexities of society, complicated technology and its scientific specialization, are all factors that cause a greater portion of our world to become more unknown and unpredictable for a greater number of people.

These circumstances can heighten anxiety to such a degree that everything signalling fear and unfamiliarity, including death, is sought erased from our personal living space, in an attempt to safeguard individual balance, that is continually threatened in our ever changing world.

Meanwhile, individual intolerance of change and the unknown varies from person to person.

Certain individuals, like anxiety neurotics, retreat painfully from even the slightest separation which might threaten their daily existence. Others, such as those with manic disorders "cast themselves about wildly in the possible" as Kierkegaard describes it, and cannot change enough. These differences, which we won't touch on here, are also important in determining the special variations which exist within the individual's repression or acceptance of death.

As Kierkegaard (1963) writes in Illness to Death, our relationship to death is closely tied up with our relationship to life, and vice versa.

If one fearfully retreats from the new and unknown in life, one will also attempt to flee from death. The need constantly to seek out continuity (non-change) is, in itself, an expression of fear of death.

It is paradoxical that, when an individual flees from his death in dread, he simultaneously loses the only chance he has of influencing death, and that possibility can change everything.

THE POSSIBILITY IN THE RELATION

For man, like all other creatures, there are some underlying, invariable and non-changeable conditions – death is one of them. But man alone is not merely determined by or identical with his conditions, in that through consciousness and reflection he can relate to them, assert himself over them, and thus simultaneously attain a significant degree of freedom in relation to these conditions.

Death isn't just a foregone conclusion, it derives its importance and effect from the individual's relationship to it. Reality is phenomenological, as the existentialists describe it.

"The glass is half empty", sighs the pessimist!

"No, the glass is half full", smiles the optimist!

The perceived is relative to the perceiver.

The glass simply "is", but it assumes its form when it meets with the subject.

It is the same with life and death. Death (or life) is neither good nor bad in the absolute – it just "is", and it is first when a person meets it – has a relationship to it – that its quality is shaped.

The fact of death cannot be changed. But through the possibilities of the relationship, man can change its content and meaning and thereby his own life as well.

Some people are so afraid to die that they don't dare live; they avoid everything new because 'what if' this or that will happen?

Death is completely absent for others - almost denied. It exists not as a personal and intensely integrated reality, but only as a theoretical abstraction that may occur some day.

This kind of person lives as if life is eternal, and in the prospective of infinity everything is indifferent, taken for granted, postponable again and again - all is levelled - and life crumbles away between his fingers without him having noticed it.

For others, death's closeness is a daily incitement. It makes every day unique and determines a genuine appreciation of being, which is only borrowed. Like the Indian Sorcerer, Don Juan, in Castenedas books, they are able to live with death sitting on their shoulder. With this perspective, life is too short to be squandered away - too important for pettiness - and too serious to not be lived responsibly. This same death (and with it, life) thus completely changes character and meaning, depending on how the individual meets it.

Every day brings each of us one day closer to our death, but no one actually knows how far away precisely the actual moment is. We all have x-number of days left to live, and these can be used in different ways from the dreadful waiting in pain of all we have to lose to the active "death on the stage".

Everything rises and falls according to which relationship is established with death, if one exists at all. "The propriety of disquiet" must, therefore, be learned so that one doesn't lose oneself by sinking into anxiety, or by never having been anxious, as Kierkegaard (1960) describes in The Condition of Anxiety.

THE ACCEPTABILITY OF ANXIETY - GROWTH POTENTIAL IN DEATH

As implied above, there is an enormous potential for development inherent in daring to become intimate with death.

Man is the only creature with the ability "to ex(s)-ist", which means to "step forward", to "stand out", to be more or less "in charge" of his own life (through the possibilities of the relationship). A thing or an animal just "is" in the world, in complete union with its nature and condition.

But as previously stated, existence is only a possibility that people have, not one to be taken for granted, and many people have trouble realizing that possibility. They live in "the figurative" (verfallenheit), as Heidegger (1960) calls it in Sein and Zeit, unaware of their specialness and the sphere of possibility in which they actually live. They therefore become like a thing, completely identified with their content, incapable of placing themselves outside it and seeing it as just one of many possible and temporary forms of existence their life can take.

Their life is, therefore, not their responsibility, and they are impersonally present without individuality, hopelessly lost in the given - in "Das Mann" - the unspecified surroundings.

Paradoxically, death and fear of death can be two of the factors which bring the individual into existence!

In the same instant that death is met as "my death", - as an anxiety filled experienced, existential reality - I am torn away from the figurative, out of "Das Mann" where death is but a collectively shared abstraction, and I become an authentic, existing person.

The closeness of death brings me into emotional contact with what the "self" that must die, and what the life I now am anxious about, actually contains and means to me. Non-being puts being into relief and thus challenges me to see the unique and irreplaceable which is myself, and to realize this before it is too late.

The anxiety that many people flee from throughout their entire life is, therefore, a basic condition for authentic life. It turns one's focus from self deception and the figurative in the world of things, back to the really important: to myself, my life, my death and my responsibility to these things!

It is, therefore, important to have the courage to be anxious! The same comprehension is seen in the Eastern philosophies.

Within Hinduism and Buddhism there is general agreement that no individual life can be meaningful and goal-orientated unless it is lived with the complete acceptance of the fact of death.

To meet death - not just as an event that awaits the end of life, but as an ever present part of the life process - is, therefore, the actual goal in both religions.

The closeness of death, like few other things, induces us to be in contact with life in a 'heartfelt' way or as Minowski (1970) writes:

"It is only in the presence of death that we come into contact in such an intimate manner with the notion of life".

It is, therefore disastrous for life to repress death. The closeness of death is what gives life intensity and authenticity.

In Catholic and Latin countries where death is physically and spiritually more present than in the Northern European and Anglo-Saxon cultures, people, as well, seem to live a more passionate and uncompromising life. One has to ask if the more muted intensity and alienated style of life that can be observed in our part of the world, has a direct connection to the collective repressions of death which is developing here. As we know, things lose their meaning and proportion in infinity. But these issues must remain open for now.

THE PSYCHODYNAMIC OF DEATH

Almost all cultures have representatives for external negative and positive energy in their religions, history, or mythology. We only have to think about our own Christian culture, where Satan and the Devil represent evil, and God or Jesus symbolize good. The Devil or God, in different disguises, assume a place in the individual, but it is first in Freud's theoretic work on instinct and management, that a systematic unravelling of aggression and the influence of the libido in the individual was made. If we are deprived, or anticipate a loss, we react with frustration which causes a mobilisation of our aggressive urge.

Man, as opposed to animals who are only capable of reacting to frustration with open aggression, has many ways of managing and channelling his frustration and aggression. This is due to his complicated psychological development, in which language plays a dominant role. It should be stressed that we refer to an unconscious, modified form of aggression, and that this is established at a very early point in human existence. For the sake of clarity, we will discuss only 4 forms of channelling of aggression. (Freud 1927 and 1946).

The first is comprised of the concept that the energy of the basic aggressive drive is unacknowledged, repressed, and thus completely absent from man's experience.

The second reveals itself in a more uncontrolled, externalized form, an aggression display with a quality of acting out.

The third canalyzing form is based upon projection. People don't acknowledge aggression in itself, but project it onto their surroundings and the surrounding people who thereby become characterized as enemies to be fought.

The fourth psychodynamic manifestation consists in introjection, the turning inward of the basic aggressive urge, and that leads to depression.

If death is regarded as life's greatest and most ultimate loss, it has to be assumed that consciousness of one's own, soon approaching death must release a very meaningful instinctual energy. These aggressive instincts, channellings, and manifestations, will change during the process of death, as described above. But the combination the individual has established in dealing with the final loss, is decisive for his quality of life and his strength in death.

An introjection of aggression means reduced quality of life, hopeless-ness, and helplessness, along with a rapid approach of death. It is as if the physical occurrence proceeds more quickly and more dramatically, when psychologically aggressive energy is introjected. Immunity is reduced, psychomotoric tempo slows down, and life energies fade away so that the physical deterioration accelerates. Realization, in itself, that the fight is lost, can cause rapid and 'incomprehensible' death in even a healthy individual.

On the other hand, it is reasonable to presume that a management of aggression which takes the form of repression and acting out, combined with consciousness of strength and happiness, not only greatly enhances the quality of life, but also demonstrably increases the length of life.

As we have already said, our mental attitude towards illness, and consequent mental intervention, is influenced by underlying, and unconscious, previously formed structures. But in as much as one is able to become aware of, modify, and change these attitudes and ways of functioning, one can give life an extra dimension, and simultaneously strengthen the quality of remaining life. (Rossi, 1986; Siegel, 1986).

OPTIMAL INFORMATION AND "THE TRUTH"

In recent years it has been emphasized that every sick person should have the right of responsibility for his own life. Since the concept "responsibility" is inextricably linked to strength and power, what we have said means that everyone has the right to have strength and power over his own life. This presupposes "optimal information" from all professional caring groups. Once and for all, we must realize that we, as Kierkegaard said, are not masters but servants, whose most distinguished duty is, through humility, understanding, and love, to discover and understand where our patient is heading, hold his hand and allow ourselves to be led.

"Optimal information" means telling the patient exactly that which he is prepared to receive. Suppression of information about the background of the disease and its development will have the effect that the patient is not provided with sufficient information for decision-making and thereby allow him responsibility for his own life. Reference can, therefore be made to the deprivation of power or strength on the therapist's part.

But, on the otherhand, "optimal information" does not mean that the patient should be told everything. Many patients don't want to know that they are approaching their death – even though most of them know it deep down. Great demands are made on the therapist's sensitivity, psychological understanding, and ethical attitudes, in order to provide the patient with information he is ready to receive, at the appropriate point. "Optimal information" has nothing to do with a finished product, which in some cases, is delivered in an attempt to soothe the therapist's conscience.

"Optimal information" is a process in which the therapist, in a close and emotional situation of trust, with sincerity, empathy, warmth and perhaps love, gently, and on the patient's terms, develops the patient's self-understanding and generates in him the strength and courage to live or die.

This information process makes further demands on the therapist's psychotherapeutic skills. How is unstated and overwhelming fear to be catalyzed? How is the patient to be comforted so that the processing of the fear isn't blocked? How does one communicate to the patient that he is not alone, but that there are 2 who bear the fear and the pain? How can a meaningless death finally be accepted in a perhaps meaningless life?

The word "truth" is a designation with modifications. First, we talk about a measurement of remaining life with a medical yardstick, which in reality can be very elastic. Secondly, some cases of so-called spontaneous remission are seen, especially in cancer patients. These are patients who have a verified and diagnosed cancer which, during a relatively short time will, ostensibly end their life, but whose condition miraculously improves when the malignant cell growth stops.

The physician's fear of telling patients "the truth" is often tied to his own fear of death which has remained unresolved. Put in another way, the physician often talks to and treats himself. He alleviates pain because it hurts him and minimizes the patient's death because he is afraid of his own death.

In the last half century of technical progress, dying has to a great extent become a technical and alienating affair, and so has life's beginning. Society's ambitious struggle to survive has made it more difficult to both give birth and to die at home. We are subject to a technical domination which gives priority to a physical shell, often at the cost of human nearness, preservation of family relationships, and understanding of the importance of psychological factors.

We have currently reached a level of research and treatment where development of the physical aspects is about to stagnate. Only a holistic attitude and a much deeper knowledge and understanding of the mind-body relationship can take us further. (Acterberg and Lowlis, 1980).

Along with man's own aggressive strength to fight death, the opposite pole – love – is the most important factor. Love is life-inducing. The love a patient cherishes for those closest to him, and the love he receives, are sources of energy in the battle against both physical and psychological decline.

Questions are many and urgent. Working with dying patients generates energy and strength to cope with our own fear of death. In these situations the therapist has a dual job. He can't just familiarize himself with and treat the patient's fear, without at the same time admitting his own anxiety and behaving accordingly. One could then perhaps conclude, that each time we work with dying patients, we lose a little bit of ourselves. In reality it's the opposite. Every time we come close to death in our daily work, our life intensity is sharpened. Only when we fully accept that death is an ever present truth in a meaningful life, will our lives gain real value, whether it lasts one day or 100 years.

REFERENCES

Acterberg, J. and Lowlis, E.F., 1980, "Bridges of the Body Mind", North Western University Press, Springfield, Illinois.
Aries, P., 1981, "The Hour of our Death", Alfred A. Knopf, New York.
Freud, A., 1946, "The Ego and the Mechanisms of Defense", International Press, New York.
Freud, S., 1927, "The Ego and the Id", Hogarth Press, London.
Heidegger, M., 1960, "Sein and Zeit", Hammeln, Copenhagen.
Kierkegaard, S., 1960, "Begrebet Angst", Gyldendal, Copenhagen.
Kierkegaard , S., 1963, "Sygdommen til Døden", Gyldendal, Copenhagen.
Minowski, E., 1970, "Lived Time", North Western University Press, Springfield Illinois.
Spengeler, O., 1923, "Der Untergang des Abendzandes", Beck, Munich.
Rossi, E.L., 1986, "The Psychology of Mind Body Healing", Harper Row, New York.
Siegel, B.S., 1986, "Love, Medicine and Miracles", Harper Row, New York.
Yalom, J.J., 1980, "Existential Psychotherapy"., Basic Book, New York.

FOUR FRAMES OF DEATH IN MODERN HOSPITAL

Anssi Peräkylä

University of Tampere
Finland

In analyzing the different perspectives on death the concept of frame developed by Erving Goffmann, is very useful. Goffmann (1974) says that the way we have framed a certain situation influences strongly on how we define that situation. Frame refers to principles of organization governing events at hand and our subjective involvement in them. Anthony Giddens (1974) follows Goffmann and says that "frames are clusters of rules which help to constitute and regulate activities, defining them as activities of certain sort and as a subject to a given range of sanctions". Frames consist of different kinds of explicit and implicit social rules, those of interpretation (constitutive rules) and normative, regulative ones. These rules make us see events around us from a certain perspective, and act respectively. As Spybey has noticed, any organization is likely to contain several frames. This is the case also in hospital.

Generally, the rules compose a very uncoherent picture about death. But when the rules are grouped as clusters, a more logical view can be attained. The clusters of rules form frames, each opening a peculiar perspective to the affairs of death and dying. The reality of death is different in each frame.

The first of these perspectives refers to the practical frame of death. Seen from this point of view, death and dying mean the set of practices enforced when somebody is dying at the ward. These practices include items like heavy nursing care, cleaning and dressing the body after the death, announcements to the family of the deceased, writing the death certificate, contacting the pathologist and so on. All different professional groups have their own tasks. The principle of organization governing the events in this frame is everyday-like means-end rationality. Everybody does her or his job following the well-earned habits trying to reach the given goal with a relatively low strain. The subjective involvement in the tasks is rather low. The rules central in this frame could be formulated like the following:

"Give primacy to everyday practical affairs when dealing with patients."

"Try to avoid dramatic scenes when dealing with patients and their families."

Besides the rules of this general type, the practical frame has as its constituents numerous rules defining in detail all the practical tasks that have to be done in the case of death.

Another frame is the biomedical one. Seen from this perspective, death and dying mean biological processes in the patient's body, which cannot be reversed by the therapeutic action. Within this frame, the central activity is to define the patient's situation in biomedical terms, and to decide the course of the therapeutic action. Diagnoses made during the life-time of the patient are usually followed by the conclusions made by physicians after reviewing the results of the autopsy. Central rules within this frame are for example the following:

"Patient's situation can and must be defined in biological and medical terms."

"Things taking place in the patient's body can and must be intervened with the help of medical facilities."

Besides the rules mentioned above, and others like them, the biomedical frame is constituted by all those interpretative rules, by the help of which physicians and nurses make their inferences about the patients' medical condition.

The third frame to be considered here is the lay frame. It is a layman's affective perspective to the affairs of death and dying. In other words, within this frame death means to the hospital staff the same as it means to people not working in hospital: an upset and existential crisis, and a call to human communion. Involvement in the dying person's situation is high, and of an affective nature. Death is accompanied by feelings of shock, anxiety, grief, and perhaps relief. Dying patient is defined as a person in need of close and intensive presence of other people. She is seen as a member of her family and the family is supposed to be emotionally upset because one of its members is passing away. Death itself is felt horribly when there is a lot of pain and ugly signs, and peaceful when the patient dies while sleeping. Among the rules constituting this frame the most central ones are like the following:

"Dying person needs presence of other people."

"It is nurses' task to be close to the dying."

"Death makes one grieve and feel bad."

"Family members are the most important people for the dying."

"Dying alone, with a great pain, and being aware of that, is horrible."

In the fourth perspective, within the semi-psychiatric frame, the issue is the experience of the patient, the family and the staff itself, constituted within the lay frame. But the involvement is dramatically different. The definitions and feelings shaped in the lay frame are now treated in a detached manner. They are interpreted and managed in terms of semi-psychiatric concepts, like repression of feelings, denial of death, acting out one's anger, and the like. The central activity within this frame is defining and controlling the tensions created within the lay frame. In this case, death means emotional processes which can be identified, controlled and managed. The central rules of this frame are like the following:

"The dying patients go through phases of different emotions when adjusting to their coming death."

"The family members of the dying patient tend to feel guilty, and that makes their demeanour sometimes strange."

"Staff members have to go through an emotional growth in order to learn to deal with the dying patients."

It is important to note that everybody participating in the dying situation - physicians, nurses, patients and their families - is acquainted with all of the above mentioned frames. The semi-psychiatric frame however, may be rather strange for a part of the patients and family members. Different groups of people have different statuses in different frames. Physicians dominate in the biomedical frame, nurses in the practical frame, and patients with their families in the lay frame. But still all understand the action within each frame, and can participate in it. For example, patients at the leukaemia ward adopt quite soon the biomedical perspective when staying in hospital. They learn to talk about the last results of different measurements made of them - also with other patients and even with their families.

The dynamics of interaction at hospital is characterized by constant shifting from one frame to another, and also by mixing the frames. Not even a short period of activity usually does take place within one frame only. Let us consider for a while the next, very usual occurrence at the leukaemia ward.

The room of an unconscious patient approaching death is attended by her husband and mother. I have joined them.	Presence of the family: Lay frame.
Two nurses come to the room, and they take a blood test from the patient. They co-ordinate their working by saying brief practical comments to each other.	Taking the blood test and talking about it: Practical frame.
When doing something to the patient, e.g. cleaning her skin or pressing the needle into her arm, one of the nurses tells, regardless of her condition, the patient what she is doing.	Talking to the unconscious patient: Semi-Psychiatric frame.
She also tells the family members what the blood is needed for: it is analyzed in order to find the bacteria in it.	Giving reasons for the blood test: Biomedical frame.
After finishing their job one of the nurses says to the family members that if they want a drink of coffee or tea, she could bring it for them.	Offering coffee as a sign of approval and encouragement for the attending family: Lay frame.

In the course of everyday activity, the different frames are laminated on each other, at each moment one of them is on the foreground, and the others are on the background.

The idea of frames makes it possible to gain a deeper understanding about the reality of dying at hospital. David Sudnow (1967) has in his excellent and by now almost classical work <u>Passing On</u> made the conclusion that death and dying mean in hospital the set of practices the hospital personnel has to engage in when somebody is dying. In the perspective opened by the notion of frames, we can easily see that this is only a partial truth. Within the practical frame death means what Sudnow says, but not within the other frames.

Same kind of comments can be made of a recent book by Anselm Strauss et al.(1985). These authors use the concept sentimental work to refer to the emotional interactions between staff and patients. They say that these kinds of interactions are participated in by the staff in order to manage and shape the patient's illness trajectories. "The many hours of conversation that nurses sometimes spend with terminally ill patients, even if enjoyed for their own sake, are designed to keep spirits up and to further the patient's closure on his or her life". Here the authors concentrate solely on the kind of orientation that I have called the semi-psychiatric frame. But besides that there is the spontaneous form of experiencing the emotional things, the lay frame. Experiencing and interaction within the lay frame could not be called work at all, although it takes place at the working place.

I think that a part of the difficulties we have in facing death in modern hospital are due to the separatedness of the four different frames and realities. Let us take two examples: the question of the intensivity of the treatment of the hopelessly ill patients, and the question of emotional response shown by the staff to the patients and their families.

I have been astonished by the amount of criticism that the staff itself directs to the active therapeutic line in the cases of hopelessly ill patients. It was almost a commonplace among the nurses to say that if I had cancer, I would never let me be treated with chemotherapy and radiotherapy as heavily as patients here are treated. Also the physicians often showed a critical attitude towards intensive treatment - although it is they them-selves who make the decisions about the care. How is it possible that the active line of treatment still goes on, when almost everybody seems to be somehow against it?

Some light to this puzzle can be attained from the conception of different frames related to death. The policy of active treatment is quite reasonable when evaluated within the biomedical frame. Within it the medical intervention into the patient's body is something taken for granted. It is within this frame that the discussion leading to the decisions on treatment usually takes place. But when nurses and physicians criticize active policies, e.g. informally talking to one and another among themselves or to the ethnographer, they act within another frame, namely the lay frame. According to the rules of this frame, death and dying are to be evaluated in terms of being horrible or peaceful. Intensive treatment obviously tends to make dying horrible.

From the above example, one can make two comments. Firstly, the example considered makes evident that different actors at hospital do not give their support to certain, coherent policies of treatment of terminally ill people. We cannot say that this doctor or nurse is for 'cure' orientation and that doctor or nurse is for 'care' orientation. In differently framed situations they all can follow and give their support for very different policies. Secondly, I want to point to the implication of the fragmented character of the social reality of hospital to the power relationships and the decision making within this institution. The fact that different frames of death are so separated from each other seems to perpetuate active policies of treatment in spite of all criticism. A hypothesis can be generalised from this: separatedness of different frames makes power immune to many potential attacks. When the attacks and their target exist in different frames, then the power attacked will not be attained by its critics.

Another problem that the staff, especially the nurses, very often face is the emotional involvement in the situation of the dying and their families. The staff's response seemed to be very ambivalent. On one hand they showed and told about strong feelings and difficulties to cope with them. On the other hand there was an evident feeling of guilt for not having enough affection. On one hand there was a strong motivation to come near to the

44

dying patient and to win her or his confidence, and on the other hand there was a tendency to keep distance between oneself and the patient.

This ambivalence can be made understandable in the light of the conception of different frames of dying. The strong feelings experienced, the affirmed obligation to have affection, and the will to be nearby the patients are responses constituted within the lay frame. The tendency towards a routinized, non emotional and distant response is constituted within the practical frame. These two responses, in spite of their logical conflict, live side by side in the world of the hospital staff. And nowadays even a third one has grown there. It is constituted within the semi-psychiatric frame, and its core is conscious management of feelings. It is needed because the feelings constituted within the lay frame are so massive, that without special management they make working very hard and tend to disturb the activities taking place in other frames.

Thus there are four different realities of death in hospital, side by side, constituted by different frames. Death means very different things in each frame. It has not always been so. In earlier times things taking place when somebody was dying could be experienced in a more holistic way. There may always have been, as Malinowski (1954) has stated, two different orientations to death, profane and practical on one hand, and sacred on the other. But these have penetrated each other: things taking place in the practical/profane domain have had their reasons and interpretations also in the sacred domain of magic and religion. In modern hospital, penetration has given way to isolation of different frames.

Dying is not at all the only phenomenon that has nowadays lost its integrity. Different authors reflecting modernization and postmodernism (see Berger et al.1973; Lyotarad, 1985) have emphasized in different terms the same thing: the over-arching discourses, or symbolic universes, have lost their power in our society. The meanings attached to experiences in different domains of life are not any more bound together. A coherent experience of the world is very hard to attain in our days. We have only partial perspectives, partial truths, on life as well as on death.

REFERENCES

Berger, B., Berger, P., and Kellner, H., 1981, "The Homeless Mind",
    Penguin Books, Harmondsworth.
Giddens, A., 1984, "The Constitution of Society", Harvard University Press,
    Cambridge, Mass.
Goffman, E., 1974, "Frame Analysis", Harvard University Press, Cambridge,
    Mass.
Lyotarad, J.F., 1985, "Tieto Postmodernissa Yhteiskunnassa", Jyväskylä,
    Helsinki.
Malinowski, B., 1954, "Magic, Science and Religion and Other Essays",
    Raven Press, New York.
Strauss, A., 1985, "The Social Organisation of Dying", Aldine, Chicago.
Sudnow, D., 1967, "Passing On: The Organisation of Dying", Prentice Hall,
    Englewood Cliffs, N.J.

VARIOUS ENVIRONMENTS SURROUNDING DEATH AMONG THE JAPANESE ELDERLY

Katsuya Inoue

Tokyo Metropolitan Institute of
Gerontology
Tokyo, Japan

It goes without saying that death is beyond the sphere of scientific recognition and cannot be understood purely on the basis of logic. Nobody can describe the experience. Death also forces us, unknowing as we are of the experience, to take leave of this world. Perhaps because of that, death has from ancient times been considered to be an unwelcome, fearsome event. The 17th century French essayist La Rochefoucauld stated that the two things that could not be doubted were the sun and death.

However, do old people, who are closer to death actually feel greater fear of it in comparison to younger people?

The results of various surveys have shown the answer to be in the negative. The survey released in 1981 by the Japanese Prime Minister's Office revealed that only 17% of elderly people in Japan were afraid of death, i.e. that the majority were not afraid of death. (Table 1)

Of course it is one thing to be afraid of death and it is another thing to talk about it to those around you. It is also possible to psychoanalytically consider that especially because death is so frightening it is kept locked deep within the unconscious in order that we don't have to feel the fear. But perhaps that is going a little too far. The reason for saying that is that if such a great repression did exist then most of the elderly would surely develop a "death fear neurosis" of some sort, but such is not in fact the case.

At the risk of being accused of throwing restraint to the winds, it is possible to say that many elderly people consider death as an established fact. If death is an established fact then the important point is not to be scared of it and try to avoid it but to decide how to accept it: how to die. Is it too much to say that most old people think of the problem as being one of a way of death?

Table 1. Frequency of subject's fear expression toward death

very often	occasional	rarely	never	others	n
3.4%	5.0%	8.6%	78.6%	4.4%	966

Table 2. Place where the elderly died

		home	hospital the elderly used to go (old)	hospital (new)	home of relatives	during the transfer	others	n
simplified overall data		49.5%	29.0%	20.3%	0.2%	0.6%	0.5%	1243
sex	♂	45.9	31.7	21.4	0	0.6	0.4	682
	♀	53.8	25.7	18.9	0.5	0.5	0.5	561
age	70–74	35.6	38.3	23.9	0	1.4	0.8	360
	75–79	49.6	28.6	20.3	0.5	0.5	0.5	409
	80–84	59.9	22.2	17.5	0.2	0	0.2	474

Based on our experience with interviews, there appear to be more elderly people who are worried about the process of dying than about itself. Most of them would rather die suddenly rather than experience a long period in a bedridden condition, or to die painlessly without any commotion. This is not evasion of the topic of death. It is in fact an approach to the topic of death.

Thus for many of the elderly, the process of dying is an important problem, yet why is this so? If there is an ideal way of death and if it can be definitely attained, then surely there would be no need to consider it as a problem. However, if this ideal cannot be attained then it would be a very great problem.

In the background to this situation of the elderly being worried about the way of dying, there are, in addition to the factor of physical pain, various other factors including psychological and social factors. I would like to consider these in the light of the results from the survey by the Prime Minister's Office.

Regardless of age or sex, for the Japanese one of the traditional ideal ways of death is to die peacefully, in one's bed on the tatami matting surrounded by an attentive family.

Let us look at the results of the survey by the Prime Minister's Office mentioned previously in which 1,243 households that had lost an elderly member were polled, to see if this is actually attained.

Table 2 shows the results of the survey showing exactly where the elderly passed away.

Looking at the simplified overall data line it can be seen that 49.5% of the elderly died at home whereas 49.3% died in hospital. In other words approximately half of the elderly were able to die lying in their bed on tatami while the other half died in hospital.

However, the elderly of course do not wish to die in hospital. This is shown clearly by Table 3. This shows the response to the question of where the elderly wish to die, based on a survey of the living elderly. Only 6% wished to die in hospital whereas, approximately 75% wished to die at home.

Taking an overview of these figures, it becomes apparent that while more than three quarters of the elderly wish to die at home, only approxi-

Table 3.　　Places where the elderly wish to die

	home	hospital	home of relatives	others	unknown
N=613	74.9%	6.2%	1.4%	0.9%	16.6%

mately half actually do so and almost all of the other half of the elderly die in a hospital, which is not where they want to die. This situation presents us with the following problem.

Death in a hospital is a fatal outcome. Nobody goes into hospital for the purpose of dying: they enter in order to cure injury or disease. Regardless of this, many old people end up dying in hospital. Therefore, regardless of whether hospitals wish this to be or not, part of their function is as an institution of death. If this be the case then in addition to the traditional role of the hospital as a place for healing and extending survival, the modern hospital takes on an added dimension as a place providing a better place to die. This means that the hospital takes on the contradictory functions as a place of healing, of extending survival and of dying, and to the extent that the modern actual facts are so, then it is impossible for us to stand idly by.

Be that as it may, hospitals, which traditionally have been places of healing and extending life, have now to take on the opposite dimension of providing a better place to die, in this case a place like home to die, for the elderly. In the future there might be two tendencies, one of the home becoming more like a hospital and the other of the hospital becoming more like home. In the case of the former, perhaps the elderly patient would be taken care of by on line monitors and other therapeutic equipment installed in his own home, or also there would be greater patient care in their own home by doctors and nurses, although there would naturally be limits to this. It would be more realistic to try to make the hospital more like home. For example in the case of a terminally ill patient who likes to drink, allowing him to have a drink, or to have favorite household articles or even in some cases a pet, allowing free visiting by friends and relatives or even permitting them to stay over. This system would be as liberal as the most liberal type of hospice in the West.

While there are still many restrictions and problems to be overcome, it would not be impossible.

Regardless, in order to try to satisfy the wish for the elderly to die at home, given the situation that most people end up dying in hospital, it will be impossible to avoid trying to solve these problems.

One of the most reassuring deaths is one in which the dying person is looked after by family or people he or she loves. On the other hand, dying alone is thought to deprive people of the courage to withstand death.

Table 4 shows the results of a survey of those present at the deaths of an elderly person. The overall data show that the dying elderly were attended by a spouse and 82.1% were attended by a child or children. In approximately 70% of cases the dying elderly person was also attended by the spouse of a child (probably the wife of a son). Thus it can be seen that more than 80% of the elderly were attended by a spouse or by their children, or both, thus the demand for a death surrounded by one's family, appears to be well satisfied.

Table 4.   People who were present at the time of death

		spouse	children	spouse of a child	grandchildren	siblings	relatives	none	n
simplified overall data		82.7%	82.1%	67.5%	36.4%	30.0%	28.1%	5.5%	1243
sex	♂	86.3	80.2	60.6	29.8	30.8	27.9	5.3	682
	♀	67.7	84.4	76.1	44.6	29.0	28.3	5.7	561
age	70–74	84.8	81.6	62.6	25.3	35.0	25.5	4.2	360
	75–79	81.4	79.2	67.2	35.9	27.6	28.5	7.6	409
	80–84	81.2	84.9	71.5	44.9	27.7	29.4	4.6	474

Table 5.   Percentage of the people who presented at the time of death and people who the elderly wanted to be present at the time of death

	spouse	children	spouse of a child	grandchildren	siblings	relatives	upper (none) lower (never want)
actual	82.7%	82.1%	67.5%	36.4%	30.3%	28.1%	5.5%
wanted	51.4	65.7	15.4	13.9	8.4	3.9	10.1

However, when one looks at the hopes expressed by living elderly concerning the people whom they wish to be attended by when they die, the satisfactory nature of the situation becomes somewhat dubious.

As is shown in Table 5, living elderly persons were asked concerning the people by whom they wished to be looked after on their death bed, and although this population was different from that on which Table 4 was based, it can be seen in all cases that there were more people looking after them than the elderly group questioned indicated they wanted. For example, 51.4% of elderly wished to be looked after by a spouse, whereas in actual fact the number of spouses attending at the death of their partner was 82.7%. What do these figures actually mean?

Although elderly persons may not express the wish to be tended to, this does not necessarily mean that they really do not want to be.

Perhaps they did not want to be tended to because of the trouble they would cause each other, or perhaps they gave up the hope, or even felt some sort of hostility to the one remaining, or perhaps they felt that the wish to be tended to was so self-evident that they did not need to express it. They might also have felt that the question was inconsequential. Thus a number of interpretations can be made, but the truth is unclear.

Nevertheless, it would be false to interpret the lack of desire for being tended to at face value. While some unsolved questions may remain, it may be acceptable to be satisfied with the high rate of family care at death.

Many people appear to be concerned with a peaceful end. A pain-filled end is perhaps the greatest threat to a human-like death.

As is shown in Table 6, a peaceful (including expression-less) death was observed in 85%, suggesting that almost all old persons are able to meet a peaceful end.

Table 6. Facial expression at the time of death

		peaceful	painful	very tense	with no expression	others	unknown	n
simplified overall data		70.6%	10.7%	1.5%	14.0%	0.5%	2.6%	1175
sex	♂	70.9	11.00	2.2	13.3	0.6	2.0	646
	♀	70.3	10.4	0.8	14.7	0.4	3.4	529
age	70–74	65.5	16.2	2.0	12.5	0.6	3.2	345
	75–79	70.1	11.4	1.9	13.8	0.3	2.6	378
	80–84	75.0	6.0	0.9	15.3	0.7	2.2	452

Table 7. Relation between frequency of painful expressions and facial expressions at the time of death

	very often	occasional	rarely	never	others	unknown	n
peaceful	14.8%	17.0%	20.3%	46.7%	0.7%	0.4%	675
painful	47.2	22.6	11.3	17.9	0	0.9	106
very tense	15.4	7.7	46.2	30.8	0	0	13
with no expression	18.8	16.2	30.8	30.8	2.6	0.9	117
others	25.0	0	25.0	25.0	25.0	0	4
unknown	28.6	4.8	9.5	47.6	9.5	0	21

However, the classification of peaceful depends on the condition at the instant of death or immediately thereafter. It is also important to understand whether the period before then, i.e. from the last time the patient went to bed until death was filled with pain or not and this is shown in Table 7.

15% of those who died "peacefully" or "with no expression" often complained of pain from the last time they were confined to bed. In other words these can be said to have been people who put an end to the pain of death. Also almost half (47.2%) of those who showed pain on death also frequently complained of pain. Thus these persons felt pain up to the moment of death and eventually died without obtaining a release from that pain.

Looking at the figures in general, while many (85%) of the elderly pass away peacefully, almost half of those (47%) complain of pain up to the end, i.e. they are people who have been released from the pain of death.

Therefore it can be seen that it is not enough to look only at the moment of death, and that it is extremely important to consider the problem of pain experienced up until the moment of death. During this period the role of pain clinics can be said to be particularly significant.

The Prime Minister's Office attempt to consider how the common wish to die peacefully, surrounded by one's family in one's own bed on tatami is being satisfied, showed clearly that the wish to die in one's own bed is not being satisfied, whether the other two categories appear on the surface to be satisfied to a large extent. However, when some of the more detailed aspects were examined it became clear that there are still some problems remaining.

The creation of an environment conducive to a better death is an extremely important and pressing problem in today's society.

THE NEST-EGG AND THE FUNERAL - FEAR OF DEATH ON THE PARISH AMONG THE ELDERLY

Ruth Richardson

Institute of Historical Research
University of London
London, U.K.

My interest in the nest-egg phenomenon has arisen from historical work on attitudes to death in modern Britain, on which I have been engaged for over a decade. This paper draws together observations made on ad hoc basis during the course of my work on related cultural phenomena. It is based mainly on data from the London area, verified by forays elsewhere and by comparing notes with others involved in oral/historical work in several other areas of Britain. I believe my work may have implications for caring practice.

Home helps, community nurses, health visitors, social workers, neighbours and other personnel caring for the elderly and the dying often find themselves taken into confidence concerning the existence of a funerary nest-egg. A sum of money has been put away to be found after the saver's death, to cover funeral costs. The money is sometimes held in a series of small insurance policies, years old, each representing small regular contributions to the nest-egg over many years. Frequently the nest-egg is in cash, and hidden somewhere in the house.

Sometimes, where there is trust between carer and saver, the confidence is shared verbally. Such occasions can take the form of a secret whispered just before death, or of an almost staged announcement to a family gathering when the saver is still alert and well. Some savers will regularly tell or remind visitors, as well as carers, in the belief that the more people who know the saver's wishes, the better the chance that the nest-egg will be found and used appropriately when it is needed. In this way, the carer is left in little doubt of the saver's intentions.

Occasionally, unforeseen events may transpire which expose the existence of the nest-egg. A stroke victim may try to fight the ambulance crew taking him to hospital until they decipher from his blurred speech that his nest-egg must go with him. A district nurse may find a nest-egg actually hidden somewhere on the body of an old lady during the course of a blanket bath. In other cases the nest-egg is found after death has occurred.

These confidences and discoverings are likely to occur wherever the elderly are cared for - whether in the community, in old people's homes, or in geriatric wards.

The cash nest-egg may represent considerable danger to the saver. Its existence is often an open secret, as cases of burglary and violence against old people bear witness. The saver's veil of secrecy may be less carefully observed by those sharing the secret, and unwise confidences may serve to promote such crimes. Funerals at the present time are so costly that a light-fingered eaves-dropper on gossip, lacking any care or appreciation of what the nest-egg represents to the old person, could find themselves tempted by tales of comparatively large sums of cash with so little to defend them. Old people have very little defence against such crimes. It is in the nature of the nest-egg's location that it must be at once hidden and yet easily found.

As old people grow to face the prospect of death, the nest-egg often becomes a locus of considerable anxiety: a fund, as it were, of complex feelings invested in its past accumulation, as well as in concern for its present preservation, and fear for its survival and rightful use. There can exist a gap of understanding between the nest-egg conserver and social and medical personnel. Colleagues and observers, even younger relatives, have been heard to express incredulity towards nest-egg behaviour - finding it by turns incomprehensible, pathetic, ridiculous or amusing. This incomprehension on the part of younger contacts and carers is probably the result of a cultural gulf between generations, or social backgrounds, and can cause misunderstanding and hurt to the elderly. I hope the materials in this paper may assist carers to understand, interpret and cope better when, in the course of their work, they encounter apparently bizarre nest-egg behaviour.

In order for us to attempt an understanding of nest-egg behaviour and the anxiety/incomprehension it may generate, two questions must be addressed: what sort of people manifest nest-egg behaviour, and why?

Who are nest-egg savers? Although cases are found in the younger elderly, nest-egg conservers are usually quite old - in their mid-seventies or older. They seem to cluster in the lower income groups, working class or lower middle class. Social origins, however, seem more influential than eventual social status. Nest-egg conservers are generally people who have experienced poverty during their formative years.

These two characteristics, considerable age and a childhood spent in poverty, indicate where we might look for some explanation of nest-egg behaviour. To understand why these people build up and conserve their nest-eggs, we must look at two related matters: first, what the nest-eggs are for; and second, what it was about growing up in poverty in the first thirty years of this century which could so have affected these people's perceptions of, and preparations for, their own demise.

What are nest-eggs for? Most people intend their nest-eggs to be used to ensure them a 'decent' funeral; that is to say, not a particularly showy or spectacular funeral, but one decent enough as funerals go. The nest-egg is a way of avoiding the indecent alternative - death 'on the parish', which nowadays means by courtesy of the social services.

Poverty and Death

People brought up in poor communities in the early decades of this century describe a culture in which death was common. Not only was there more death about, but poor children were more likely to be exposed to it in the culture in which they were reared. It was amongst the poor and working class that traditional observances associated with death survived the longest. (Richardson, 1976)

Preparation for death has long been an important element in traditional observance. In the 1920's one writer recorded that old women 'forced by circumstances to spend their last days in the workhouse, take with them a nightdress and a pair of white stockings in order that they may appear 'respectable' at their death' (Puckle, 1926). 'Like many an old working class woman,' writes Richard Hoggart, 'my grandmother had a splendid laying-out gown and sheets ready against her death, and towards the end of her life she would remind us periodically where they were kept' (Hoggart, 1959). Though the custom is now comparatively rare, considerable care is taken even today by some old women to have their burial-clothes clean and ironed, and put away safely. As a child, one of my respondents (born in 1901) was given a traditional shroud by her grandmother, in case she grew up to die in childbirth. She still has it, and proposes to use it when her time comes.(1) In the early years of this century, the keeping of the customary shroud and white stockings within poor homes would have been known even to small children, who often observed the custom of visiting the corpses of recently deceased family members, friends or neighbours.

Financial preparation for death was also customary. In the early years of the century an important survey asked women subsisting on a wage of about £1 a week to keep accounts of their budgets. A recurring characteristic of these meagre budgets was that the women who kept them regularly spent five to ten percent of their weekly income on death insurance. In these years, the level of anxiety surrounding saving for death was very high. Death insurance was called the 'one great universal thrift of the poor'. Why was this the case?

First, the economic reasons. A death, even of a child, could economically devastate a poor family. There could be no margin of solvency on a low income to pay for a decent funeral, which could cost anything from four to ten times an average male weekly wage. There were no safety nets to support a poor family other than the feared and hated workhouse. Death could both bereave and pauperize. Maud Pember Reeves (1913) referred to the 'horrible problem' constantly faced by the poor: unless regular insurance payments were made for every member of the family; at death there was no other prospect than that they should each face disposal as a pauper, or pauperize the family.

The desire not to inflict financial hardship on survivors, not to be a financial burden at death, is a characteristic feature of nest-eggers with surviving family and friends. Their disposable property is generally meagre, and of little value. Most people who prepare to leave a nest-egg have no solicitor, and generally, no written will. Those utterly alone in the world have no other way to express a will. The nest-egg is the material manifestation of the saver's will. It represents independence, self-containment and a final part of putting one's house in order before death. It also represents a moral imperative to survivors, be they family or not, to respect the saver's wish for a decent funeral.

The Fear of The Pauper Funeral

Throughout the Victorian era, and well into the twentieth century, the fear of the pauper funeral has afflicted the British poor and working classes. What we see now among some of the elderly is the survival of these attitudes into our own time. Wilson and Levy (1939), investigators of death insurance during the Great Depression of the 1930s, reported: 'the present effect of the pauper burial is of much greater significance (than the emulation of social superiors) for its avoidance is considered a dire necessity, and constitutes the stimulus which drives people to enter life policy agreements, however ill they can afford it.

The calculated indignity of the pauper's funeral dates from the early 19th century, when public expenditure on poverty was cut by the New Poor Law.

_____

(1) My respondent Mrs W., born 1901, West London.

Those who failed to provide for themselves in life were taken to the workhouse. Those who failed to provide for themselves in death were taken to
their long home naked, wrapped only in paper, or a strip of calico stretched
over the corpse. Coffins were of the cheapest possible materials and standards of workmanship, made of the thinnest wood, often unplaned, and instead
of a lining, a layer of sawdust. Relatives were denied the customary farewell 'last look' and had no say in when or where the burial might take place.
The journey to the burial ground was hasty and careless. Pauper graves were
dug in land attached to the local workhouse, or in the most neglected parts
of local burial grounds. The graves themselves could be twenty or more
coffins deep, all generously treated with quicklime to hasten speedy re-use.
A number would invariably be the only indication of the space in which
generations of workhouse and parish poor were laid: no monument marked a
pauper's grave.

   The pauper funeral was thus an exemplary mode of disposal, an object
lesson to all. It was a beacon of 'social worthlessness, earthly failure,
and profound anonymity' (Laquer, 1983). As one Manchester respondent put it;
"a pauper funeral was the failure of your life". (2)

   What we may encounter today as a curious attachment to a collection of
money, or an incomprehensible wish for a decent funeral may often be the
residue of the memory of these indignities. For although fear of death on
the parish eased somewhat with the advent of the Death Grant and the Welfare
State, the elderly often carry with them an awareness of the disgrace which
attached to pauper burial in their parents' and grandparents' generations.
Although most of my own interviewees had never actually seen a pauper's
funeral, the indignity involved was notorious by repute. "It was terrible
to have to be buried by the parish - that's why we all had insurance." (3)
One of my respondents described a pauper funeral he had seen in Marylebone,
London, just before the Great War: they used to have a baby's hearse, where
the little coffin went under the driver's seat, well, in a pauper's funeral,
they used to push the big coffins under the seat - and the ends used to stick
out. (4) The intention seems to have been publicly to humiliate and vilify
the dead and their family for having failed to keep up insurance payments
or somehow to find the money for a decent funeral. Although this particular
form of humiliation seems to have been a practice peculiar to Marylebone in
these years, it was of course in every undertakers' interest to render
burials conducted on behalf of the parish as undignified as possible: the
perpetuation of the stigma would perpetuate the endeavour to avoid it, which
would of course promote more lucrative business.

   A change in public attitudes towards poverty, and the greater profess-
ionalism of undertaking has made a such a deliberately undignified spectacle
unlikely today. Yet parish funerals, or 'contract' funerals as they were
known in the trade, still offer only the barest essentials, and conform to
their slang names - the 'nine o'clock trot' - since they are generally
undertaken early in the morning. Parish coffins are usually the cheapest
unvarnished chipboard. As one undertaker explained to me, "an undertaker
can only give a minimum service ... because, em, it would be unfair in truth
to do otherwise; because people who were paying for a - shall we say - a
funeral conducted in the normal way, they would in fact be subsidizing the
other. (5)

   There are also darker elements in the fear of parish burial. The
elderly today probably have little more than a residual notion of precisely

---

(2) Respondent recorded in Manchester by Audrey Linkaan.
(3) My respondent Mrs W., born 1901, West London.
(4) My respondent Mr R., born 1898, Marylebone, Central London.
(5) My respondent Mr A., undertaker, born 1920, South London.

what it was that their parents and grandparents regarded with such horror; but folk memory reverberates down generations. The Victorian pauper burial counted among its more regular components – paper shroud, flimsy coffin, dose of quicklime and unmarked grave – something even more sinister. The Victorian poor also knew that death in poverty could mean that appropriation of the corpse for dissection. Formerly, for centuries, dissection had been a judicial aggravation of the capital punishment for murder; but in 1832 it was transferred to poverty by the widely unpopular Anatomy Act, administered locally by the Poor Law authorities. The fact that the misfortune of a death in poverty could qualify a person for dismemberment after death was an intensely painful element in fears of parish disposal. (6)

A similar and more modern element is the general awareness that the corpses of those disposed of by the parish today are usually cremated. Although voluntary cremation accounts for over 50% of all deaths today, and although many people generously bequeath their bodies to science, there is still considerable repugnance to being burnt or dissected after death, particularly if this is against one's will during life.

Historically, the nest-egg can therefore be seen as a poor person's only defence against being disposed of in such ways. It is the only way in which a poor person can register their wish for a decent disposal after death. The nest-egg is their only insurance that their wishes during life will be observed in death.

REFERENCES

Hoggart, R., 1959, "The Uses of Literacy", Harmondsworth, London.
Laquer, T., 1983, Bodies, death and pauper funerals, in Representations
    Vol.1(1)109.
Puckle, B., 1926, "Funeral Customs", London.
Reeves, M. P., 1913, "Round About a Pound a Week", London.
Richardson, R., 1976, Death in the Metropolis, unpublished.
Wilson, Q. and Levy, H., 1939, "Industrial Assurance", London.

---

(6) I trace the history and social meaning of the Anatomy Act in my
    forthcoming book, "Death, Dissection and the Destitute" (in preparation)

TERMINAL CARE IN CHILDREN

Elspeth Brewis

Royal Hospital for Sick Children
Glasgow, U.K.

Terminal care is that which prepares someone for death. Preparation should start at the diagnosis of a potentially fatal disease, or when active, curative treatment is acknowledged to be no longer appropriate. Treatment is therefore changed to an equally positive one that aims for a "good death".

In an ideal world children would not die; it can be quite a shock to realise that they do. Although probably a fifth of child deaths are sudden where preparation is impossible (such as accidents - most of which are road traffic accidents - burns, falls, poisonings, inhalations, sudden infant deaths etc.); for the majority of deaths there is the opportunity for some preparation, if only briefly (this group includes neonatal deaths, infective diseases, meningitis, acute-laryngobronchitis etc). Those with chronic disorders, where preparation time could well be counted in months or even years, include muscular dystrophy, multiple handicaps, congenital abnormalities, renal or cardiac disorders, cystic fibrosis, and cancers - these last being the largest single cause of deaths after accidents. There is a strong impression among paediatric nurses within the U.K. that more and more children are dying at home rather than in hospital.

The decision to stop active treatment can be quite devastating to parents; the fact that death might be inevitable does not necessarily make it easier to accept. The fact that their aspirations for their child's future will not reach realisation is hard, if not impossible, to grasp ultimately. The decision to change therapy is reached after much discussion between the hospital team (which has probably instigated care up to the present) and the parents. The explanations are that curative treatment has failed, the progress of the disease cannot be halted, and there should be a change to positive palliative care.

Parents need reassurance that pain etc. will be controlled, and that they won't be 'deserted', and that support will be ongoing. The more preparation and discussion that goes into such a decision the easier it is for the professionals, as well as the parents, to believe that the decision made was the right one; the parents have to live with the decision all their lives. Yet we must not remove hope entirely.

The devastation of the isolation felt by parents at this point can almost seem like a bereavement in itself. They feel they are on their own - the safety of the hospital and all its support has been taken from them -

during the preceeding months (or years) the hospital and staff have become their world. It is a bit like the rubber ring being taken away when you haven't yet learnt to swim. At this point even the staff feel devastated – 'we have failed, we are guilty, and our hopes too are dashed'. But we should not hide how we feel, because like it or not, we are all in it together – we too had the same aspirations of cure at first, why else did we become involved?

Once the decision is taken to change treatment it may be that the child has a 'lot of living to do' (as can be the case in a child with relapsed cancer). If the condition/state of health allows there is no reason why that special holiday or activity should not be undertaken. However, common-sense must prevail and crises anticipated, for example, carrying a covering letter to the nearest casualty department in the event of sudden treatment being needed.

Support for the parents is extremely important – after all, whether in or out of hospital, they are the primary care-givers – and this means reassurance that all will be done to help, not just at the end of a tele-phone one hopes, but with professionals having time to sit and listen. In order that this can be the best that can be provided, inter-disciplinary communications must be honest, accurate, frequent and ongoing. Within hospital this should be relatively easy, but the hospital does not satisfy all the medical, nursing and social needs. Doctors should communicate with the general practitioner as early as possible. The more confident the community doctor is in knowing what is and has been going on the better will he be able to support the family. This could well be his first experience of caring for a dying child at home, and it will be a very difficult situa-tion for him on a personal level as well as a professional one.

The same is true of the community nursing service. They could be invited to the hospital to discuss the problems, treatment, and expectations with colleagues, or at least meet a member of the nursing team, maybe in the home of the child; it is so much easier to communicate with someone who already knows something of what has gone before. If one walks into a home as an unknown one feels helpless, and although not so, the feeling of inadequacy is difficult to overcome.

Wherever a child is finally nursed is usually the parents decision. It is probably true to say that all families cope better than expected when it comes to terminal care, and it is insulting for professionals to say 'they couldn't cope' – it is up to them to ensure that the family does. It is the role of all involved professionals to provide all the physical, material and emotional support and guidance they can. Throughout the terminal illness life goes on, and activities such as play, in any form that can be indulged in, must be readily available, and schooling too! One is aiming for the best quality of life.

If the child is to die in hospital, there should be little problem with communications as everything and everyone is 'on tap', dieticians, occupa-tional therapists, physiotherapists, teacher, etc. etc. who all have a role to play. The parents should be able to do as much of the care as they are able and willing; they know the child better than anyone, and are best able to meet his needs, likes, foibles, and habits. Participation for them is, in a way, therapeutic – they need to believe, after the child's death that "we did everything we could". Being resident in hospital if possible is very helpful to all. Family and friends should freely visit with the agreement of everyone (space and sheer numbers of persons within the ward could be limiting factors). As many personal things as can reasonably and safely be accommodated from home should be allowed. The 'terminal state' should not prevent children being allowed outside, in a car, pram/pushchair, anyhow into the fresh air, or to the museum or whatever is available, as it allows child and carers to be together in a different environment, even if temporarily, and it is good for everyone. There are no hard rules, just flexibility. The advantage of hospitalisation is the number of people around and available to offer support. The disadvantage is that it can happen that everyone thinks that someone else is providing the support when each professional is rushing from one urgent task to another! One way round this situation is the Primary Nurse - she it is who co-ordinates care. She should ideally be a qualified nurse who has been involved with the family over some considerable time, is familiar with the care given in the past, and is aware of the present and able to plan for the future. Parents must always realise that they can change their minds and take their child home if they wish.

If the child is to die at home, it may be difficult for some members of the family group to come to terms with a dying child at home, some may wish to deny what is going on (it may be a part of the way they cope), and perhaps not be able to watch the child deteriorate (that is, become less active, thinner/fatter, paler, restless, perhaps in pain, and 'demanding' (ie. needing more attention). Some may feel that they could not face the event without the protection of the hospital 'coccoon'. At home the co-ordinating nurse, the Primary Nurse, will be a community nurse.

Such a tragedy as the death of a child is a family event and cannot be hidden - the siblings, even the very young, will remember this event all their lives, therefore how it is handled is very important - feeling 'left out' is a very bitter feeling, and cannot easily be undone. The big advantage of the home environment is that normality has a better chance of existing, with all one's own things around. The opportunity for the family to be together is higher, and the opportunity for free family communications is there. Having said that, it can be that this situation is the breaking point between parents. The chronic illness of children so often causes either a greater bond between parents, or the very opposite, as the sick child demands so much of the mother's time and attention. Therefore there is a great need to ensure that the parents too are cared for. This could mean simply ensuring that they eat properly, get a good night's sleep sometimes, are helped with shopping, or baby-sitting. Allowing the parents time together provides a few precious moments for them to share feelings and worries, as it is all too common for parents to be unable to communicate adequately, as they do not see themselves as important. However, as time goes on the parents hold the time left with their child very jealously and come to a stage when they will not allow anyone else to do any caring nor leave the child at all; they fear the coming of the moment which will have been the last.

Symptom control becomes the most important aspect of care, and often the hardest, as some symptoms are very tricky to solve, for nurses are practical people, and they like to be doing things if they can! The variety of problems may well depend upon the original diagnosis, and 'more of the same' may be indicated, eg. more anticonvulsant therapy even if it makes the child sleepier, more oxygen and antibiotics to help the laboured breathing, more baclofen to control muscular spasm, more radiotherapy to relieve pain or disfigurement of those suffering from some form of cancer. It may mean naso-gastric feeding to alleviate thirst, a most distressful symptom. Vomiting may be intractable for some diagnoses; previously successful anti-emetics may cease to be effective, yet other, long discarded, may come into their own again - there is so much trial and error, but constantly striving to improve the status quo must be the greatest motivator.

Ensuring a good nights sleep may mean sedatives; antibiotics might be indicated to remove the distress of some infection. Pain control is the hardest - it is so difficult to assess pain, even listening to the child

and the parent. If the child says he has pain, then he has, but how to
solve it is the tricky bit. For some, Paracetamol might be all that is
needed, for others a combination of MST or Diamorphine along with a tran-
quiliser may be the only things that 'touch it'. Increasingly the use of
a syringe driver is proving beneficial - except that those who have had to
cope with endless injections in the past might not readily tolerate the idea
of this method of giving analgesia. The main thing is to see that analgesia
is readily available, and leaving a tablet out for the child to give himself
at night (so that he need not disturb his parents) might be appropriate at
home, and a positive step for the adolescent, who can have some degree of
control on his own care. One must also always be alert to the simple things,
which can so easily be overlooked in the anxiety of the complexity of the
situation.

Although the child is fiercely individual, each child is an integral
part of a family, whatever its size, each member of which has needs that
require consideration. Any physical separation need not mean an emotional
separation.

The child's understanding of what is going on varies with his age and
stage of development (the finality of death develops with age), his comprehension of life and death, eg. the understanding of a child who has lost
a favourite grandpa or dog will be more mature than that of a child of the
same age with no experience, and his diagnosis. For example, a child with
cystic fibrosis is usually very 'au fait' with his disease, prognosis and
outcome - he has "seen it all" with his fellow sufferers. As with the child
with cancer he knows who comes to the clinic at the same time and he notices
the gaps. Sometimes youngsters go to funerals of others. An honest response
to the question of "where is ......?" is given, and frequently offered when
one is aware of a particular friendship between children or parents.
Children are used to honest answers (or should be), but sometimes courage
fails the parents - a 12 year old was aware that a 3 year old fellow patient
had died (and not been moved elsewhere as he had originally been told by his
mother). When a couple of months later he enquired of the whereabouts of
another child he was given the same story as before, that the child had been
moved. He said "are you telling me the same lie you told me before?".
Ultimately this mother was glad that before it happened, she and her son
were able to talk about his own death.

Children do ask questions, and sometimes lots of them (as they do when
well, like "why is the Clyde called the Clyde?"). "Can I go and visit my
wee brother (in heaven) and then I'll go to the party?". "Does it hurt to
die?" - one hopes not. "Am I going to die?" - well, we all do sometime,
and no one knows just when, but what makes you feel that you might die? are
you frightened? One should stay for comfort and make oneself available for
further questions or discussion. Such questions and the responses given,
must be forwarded to the parents, so that the handling of that child may be
consistent - there is no point one person denying death, if another has just
said that we all die, some sooner rather than later. We should never presume
that we understand the thought behind the question, it could be one entirely
different from our own, so it is vital to clarify the question before
answering. "I think I'm dying" said a child, "what ever makes you say that"
enquired nurse, "I've got a tummy-pain, and my mummy says that she's dying
when she has a tummy-pain". We should not jump to conclusions; receiving
a reply you are not expecting to a serious question can give rise to added
confusion. (This is also true when responding to adults). "Where is
heaven?" - good question. "Sister, do you want to hear a joke? I'm going
home today with my drip!" (teehee!) He died that day.

It can happen that a child does know his diagnosis and its implications,
yet his parents be unaware of this, and sometimes children do not want their

parents to know that they know, (and this is not just so with the older teenagers). A similar protective mechanism as seen between spouses can arise – the child senses (probably has done for a long time) that the subject of his illness upsets his parents, so he will not ask questions of them. "Don't cry, Mum, I'll be alright, I'll be good".

Fear in a child shows in differing ways; asking no questions, saying nothing, asking everything 10,000 times, complaining of some non-existant problem, or saying "I want my Mummy" when she is sitting right beside him! A child's memory of pain is relatively short – if he doesn't have one he doesn't brood in case he does have one (usually), but mention the word 'jag' and he soon remembers! Teddy can provide a useful communication tool in the very young child; one takes both sides of the conversation expressing anxieties using teddy to help with the replies. This is fine until one touches on things that are very private when teddy will be pulled away from the conversation. He (or rather the child) has had enough.

The most junior nurse is especially vulnerable. Apart from her own very delicate feelings, she is readily available for the unexpected and difficult questions, as she seems not to be hampered by authority and its implied inaccessibility. "I don't want to bother Sister, but could you tell me .....?" At least the junior nurse has the advantage of saying truthfully 'I don't know, I'll go and ask', and then she must return with an answer, even if it is also 'I don't know, but I'll find out'. It might well have taken courage to ask the question in the first place so it should be respected and given a response. Most questions have answers, and it is difficult to accept that sometimes there is no answer, not even from the priest/minister. The response 'we must wait and see' has only a limited use if one is the questioner.

One should not make promises that one cannot keep, eg. 'this is your last injection' – all too often the course of therapy changes, and the best method of symptom control might be an injection of some sort. Everyone should tell the same story, therefore communications between staffs, parents, etc. is vital, and they must be accurate and consistent. If anyone thinks that they might have 'put their foot in it' and said something they should not, they must admit it to a professional who can deal with it, right the wrong, soften the blow, or sort out the confusion.

If someone expresses a worry, (be it patient, parent or nurse) one should readily admit that they are entitled to worry. We all know how easy it is to say 'don't worry', yet find it difficult to 'not worry'. There is no such thing as being 'over-anxious' – there are no Permitted Levels of Anxiety – if a parent seems to have an inappropriate anxiety then the carers should consider that they are not dealing with the problem, which probably needs more time and patience.

We all want recovery for a sick child, but need to admit to ourselves that this can be an unreal expectation. That does not mean that we have the right to deny hope to the parents (or the child) and yet remain honest. There are no guarantees in the game of life. We all wish the inevitable would not happen. One four year old desperately wanted something: "But I WANT it!" she said, 'You don't say 'I WANT' – how do you ask for something nicely, what is the magic word?', I expected to hear the word 'please'. "ABRACADABRA!" came the very solemn reply – I wish that that was the solution to all our problems!

TERMINAL CARE IN THE OLD

Clifton Lowther

Royal Victoria Hospital
Edinburgh, U.K.

Only 24% of the population die before the age of 65 and Table I shows the distribution of death in 10 year groups therafter. My starting point is therefore that most dying is done by the old and therefore it is appropriate to study their deaths perhaps more than has been done in the past. Isaacs and his colleagues (1972) looked back retrospectively from the deaths of old people in the West of Scotland and examined the pre-death phase. He elaborated the idea of "pre-death" as being a period during which physiological functions were maintained by an inherent medullary programme long after any recognisable person had disappeared. Fries and Crapo (1981) extrapolated from past successes in pushing morbidity and mortality into later life and proposed that there would eventually be a time when the expectation of life would approximate to the span of life and that we would all depart after a relatively short, sharp illness. There has been quite widespread criticism of this optimistic concept. In fact however very little has been written about the length of the period of decline and dependency terminating in death in the old. My comments are directed towards consideration of death in people on the far side of 75 years and mainly on the far side of 80 years of age. Perhaps I should give you some rather black good news. Amongst the old 10% fall down dead; less than 2% experience what has been described as the horrors of the geriatric long stay ward and the rest of us die reasonably quickly and tidily after quite a short final illness.

Table 1. AGE AT DEATH (Scotland 1985)

Age	64	65–74	75–84	85+
Deaths (Percent)	24%	25%	32%	19%

Table 2. LIVING ALONE (Household Survey 1985)

Age	45–64	65–74	75+
Percent	10.4%	28%	47%

Table 3. WHAT WE DIE OF

	45 – 74 years	75 years +
CIRCULATION	44 – 50%	60%
NEOPLASM	25 – 30%	13%
RESPIRATORY	12 – 16%	17%
ETC	4 – 8%	10%

In what way does death in the old differ from the deaths more usually considered in writings on terminal care? In the first place death is not seen as the enemy to be resisted at all costs but only the last of a series of losses which have been experienced by the old, over a period, the loss of the mate, the loss of friends, the loss of contact with the society in which one lives, are a few of these inevitable losses experienced by the old before death. Death, in a word, is not premature and therefore not necessarily an unwelcome guest. Death is seen by the old as appropriate with acceptance rather than mere resignation. "I have lived long enough" and it is with some difficulty that one restrains younger professionals from making an immediate diagnosis of severe depression. The old in fact are much more concerned with possible discomfort and loss of dignity and privacy, particularly during the pre-death period, than they are with the ultimate end, and even the hereafter. I should perhaps say, as an agnostic bystander in this area that religion seldom seems to enter into the ultimate phase except amongst the attendants who are still at a stage in their lives when they have a good deal to thank their God for. Advice to the old during the later phases of life is strangely thin on the ground from those who might be expected to contribute, namely, philosophers, sociologists and ministers of religion. What is offered is only the bleak prospect noted by Robert Burns "For we Maun totter doon John and hand in hand we'll gae". This is not even epidemiologically correct as John's hand along with the rest of John is usually underground for a considerable part of his widow's late life.

Death in the old is more likely to take place in an institution because they are more likely to be living alone. Table 2 shows the proportion of persons living alone in the UK as age increases. As they are more likely to be living alone their final illness and death are more likely to take place in an institution than they are in earlier age groups. It must be remembered that amongst those 80 years and over in this country, something like a fifth never had any children and a further 18% only ever had one child. Amongst other factors this increases the likelihood of aloneness at the latter end. Apart from family size, other unavoidable factors contribute to the loneliness of the aged, namely, mobile population, smaller houses, old age pensioner and sheltered housing which are divisive, occasionally rejection but mainly of course the preference of the old for living by themselves, close to but not necessarily with their children.

Death in the old is more likely to be a resultant of many factors than it is in the elderly or earlier age groups and the certification of the cause of death in the old is notoriously inaccurate. From Table 3 it can be said that a gradient exists in what is recorded as the cause of death but in fact all that one can say is that the old are likely to die with circulatory disease, with neoplasm or with respiratory disease rather than of any one of these diseases. It is much more likely in earlier life that one single disease process can be pinpointed as the cause of death, but it should also be remembered that whatever the disease the old may have, these exist on the basis of a body with significantly impaired homeostatic mechanisms and organ reserves. From the foregoing it is clear that the direction of diagnosis, investigation and symptom management is much more complicated in the old than it is in earlier age groups, less clearly defined by the attendants and by implication, more likely to be accompanied by inappropriate medical and nursing management. Thus, multiple pathology leads to multiple pharmacy which leads to multiple side effects which leads to even more drugs. All this further complicates the diagnostic, clinical and prognostic picture.

The quality of life assumptions in the terminal phase in earlier age groups are more likely to approximate to those of the attendants and relatives and therefore likely to be those of younger, possibly richer persons more in charge of their own destinies and probably more motivated by philanthropic and (recently) defensive elements in their approach to these problems. In age the quality of life cannot be assessed on behalf of the patient even if they are consultable, except possibly by those with long experiences in this area of work who are willing and able to spend much time being with and listening to the dying. In my opinion there is no harm in quality-of-life value judgements if you have to make them on behalf of unconsultable patients. The important point is to know that you are making a value judgement and not pretend that it is a scientific one. Everyday a new scale or index is elaborated to add to the Sickness Impact Profile, the Life Satisfaction Index, the Quality of Well Being Index, The Visual Linear Analogue Scale, the Anxiety/Depression Scale, the Quality Adjusted Life Years Calculation, the Philadelphia Geriatric Morale Scale, the Society Adequacy Scale, the Sorle Morale Scale, the Zung Self Rating Scale, the Death Anxiety Scale and the Minnesota Multiphasic Personality Inventory. After participating in only a few of these the old might well feel death was a merciful release.

Because of the presence of multiple pathology on a basis of involutionary changes in the body and mind, there is liable to be a longer period of decline in the pre-death phase amongst the old than there is amongst the younger age groups. It is therefore more difficult to answer the question "when is dying?" and to delineate clearly therefore the important water-shed which separates the period of therapeutic optimism from the period of positive "settling for comfort".

The relationship to relatives is also different in age. In early life the relatives are the parents. In middle life the relatives are the peers. In late life they are occasionally the aged mate but more often the children. There are therefore obvious difficulties in communication and consultation which are peculiar to the aged as they are much less part of a family scene, being much more isolated long distance runners. They depend for the maintenance of their rights and their wishes more on their relationship with their attendants than with their relatives, especially as at present they are more likely to be dying away from home. There are clearly unique difficulties in consulting children about the terminal management of their parents. Consultation is also difficult however, in certain groups of patients. In the care of the old when the dying phase appears to be with us, the patients tend to divide themselves for practical management purposes into 3 groups. First are those who have retained mental capacity and personality although often suffering from very severe physical disabilities. Such people are totally consultable and if a good meaningful relationship has been created between them and their attendants they can be consulted on what it is that they think should happen e.g. with reference to decisions about surgery or invasive diagnostic procedures. There are then patients who are dying with physical disease but also some measure of dementia which makes meaningful consultation impossible. Their personalities are retained, however, and management then depends on one's objective estimate of how much they are still attached to life as shown by interest in relatives, neighbours and improved health as well as by demonstration of anger, or the wish to choose and decide. Even under the poor long-stay circumstances some old people in this group still want to see what happens tomorrow. The third group is a good deal more of a problem, namely those dying with a great burden of physical disease and mental impairment with no communication or

consultation possible, and it is here that the most anxious decisions fall
to be made by the attendants. Younger attendants are frequently overly
insistent on the mere continuation of life which arises from their own
insufficient self knowledge and from their insufficient knowledge and experience of the cogitations and life considerations of the old. The young
have little understanding and often little sympathy with the life of the old
because it is difficult to think yourself into a life in which ambition,
fame, passion, getting and spending and even outside interests have contracted down or actually disappeared.

The problems which present themselves at this time are not necessarily
the common one of whether or not to prescribe an oral antibiotic in what
might be a terminal chest infection but the much more difficult considerations of how to deal in unconsultable seriously damaged and deteriorated
patients with persistent gastro-intestinal bleeding, peripheral gangrene,
a painless perforation of an abdominal viscus, major fractures or the onset
of total dysphagia from stroke. These are the kind of difficulties in which
the age and background condition of the patient become paramount when
deciding future management and in which in the course of my last 25 years
in Geriatric Medicine I found myself making mistakes both of commission and
omission. At an earlier point, and in the area of preventive medicine there
is also the question of whether to innoculate unconsultable patients against
influenzal pneumonia in a closed ward community when many would regard onset
of such a illness as being a consummation devoutly to be wished. What is
important is that if it is accepted that these major medical and surgical
problems are not going to be actively and radically pursued then the
attendants must accept fully the need for adequate relief from distress,
really regardless of the limitations of the standard pharmacopeia.

Finally, as we have seen over the centuries and decades, the old and
the sick and dying move progressively out of the prestigious voluntary
hospitals into local authority hospitals and which in their turn become
prestigious and wish to move such patients on. Much of this care has
gravitated to primary care and geriatric units. Of late, however, geriatric
medicine itself which has long provided the humane caring required by this
age group is now beginning to talk about "high turnover", of "short packages
of rehabilitation" and of more recently of "performance indicators". Once
again I fear that the old and dying with multiple incurable diseases are on
the move, perhaps back to their own homes.

REFERENCES

Fries, J. F., and Crapo, L. M., 1981, "Implications of the Rectangular
    Curve", Freeman, San Francisco.
Isaacs, B., 1972, "Survival of the Unfittest", Routledge and Keegan Paul,
    London.

RISK FACTORS ASSOCIATED WITH MORTALITY AMONG THE ELDERLY BEREAVED

Ann Bowling

Institute for Social Studies in Medical Care
London, U.K.

INTRODUCTION

Mortality rates for widowed people are known to be higher than those for married people. The excess risk is greater for men than women (Bowling and Benjamin, 1985).

Various hypotheses have been forwarded in attempts to explain this. These have focused on the physical and mental impact of the stress of bereavement, reduced social support and the difficulties of taking on new roles (Bowling, 1968).

There is a physical and psychological basis for the excess risk of mortality among the widowed, and widowers in particular. The widowed consult doctors more often, take more medication and have generally higher symptom and illness rates than the non-widowed (Maddison and Viola, 1968; Parkes and Brown, 1972; Bowling and Cartwright, 1982). The evidence suggests that widows report more acute illnesses and widowers report more chronic problems (Carter and Glick, 1976; Bloom, Asher and White, 1978; Gove and Hughes, 1979). In addition, widowers have also been found to take longer than widows to recover from depression following bereavement (Parkes, 1975).

There is little research investigating the relationship of the social, psychological and physical characteristics of the bereaved with the duration of their survival following bereavement. This is because representative samples of widowed people are difficult and expensive to obtain.

THE SURVEY

A national study of the elderly widowed was carried out by myself and Dr Ann Cartwright. This study was based on interviews in 1979 with a national random sample of elderly people who had been widowed for about 5 months. This survey provided the sampling frame for a subsequent study of mortality rates after bereavement.

The rationale of the initial sampling procedure, response rates and methods have been described in detail in 'Life after a Death'. A study of the elderly widowed (Bowling and Cartwright, 1982). A total of 503 people, mostly over retirement age, who had been widowed in January (a few in late

December) 1979, were sampled randomly from the death certificates of their
spouses. About three quarters of these were successfully interviewed and
proxy interviews were held with carers of a further 4% who were too ill to
be interviewed. Fifteen people had died before we could interview them (3%),
2% had moved and were untraced and 20% were unwilling to talk to us, despite
a repeated request at the end of the interviewing period. Some of these
said it was too upsetting to talk about the death.

The interview survey was a descriptive study of the lives of the widowed
people. The measures used, and which were analysed in relation to mortality
for the follow up, included measures of health status, social support and
involvement, emotional adjustments and wellbeing.

The initial sample of 503 widowed people (responders and non-responders)
was entered into a prospective flagging operation by the Office of Population
Censuses and Surveys.

The aims of the flagging were to document the widowed's mortality rates
and to analyse these, for responders, in relation to the information collected in 1979 about their social, psychological and physical characteristics.

The hypothesis to be tested was that low levels of social support and
poor emotional wellbeing would be associated with increased risk of mortality
after bereavement.

RESULTS

In the six years between January 1979 and January 1985, 25% of the widows
and 38% of the widowers had died - that is, over a quarter (29%) of the
initial sample of 503.

Death rates were lower among the 361 responders, 24% compared with 38%
of the 123 non-responders (this includes the 15 who died before the interview), and 58% among the 19 frail widowed for whom we obtained proxy interviews.

Comparison of the mortality rates of the total sample (of responders and
non-responders) with those of the total population of the same ages, by sex,
was made using the Registrar General's Life Tables for England (Bowling and
Benjamin, 1985).

For widowers and widows, aged under 75, mortality rates were no different
from those of men and women generally. However, for men aged 75 or more
there was evidence of excess mortality in the first six months of bereavement
(t-test:$P<0.05$). There were twice as many deaths among males aged 75+ as
would be expected in the general population of males of the same ages. The
mortality rate for females aged 75+, however, was lower than expected.

Bi-variate analyses using X2 tests showed relationships with mortality
and having a low level of social contacts, a low level of emotional wellbeing
and with taking a greater amount of non-psychotropic medication (there was
no relationship with mortality and self reported health status and functional
ability). These relationships were generally stronger for males and for the
widowed aged 75+.

Logistic regression analysis was used to explore the relationship between
these characteristics and mortality, while holding the effects of age and sex
constant. All two-way interactions, involving age and sex, were tested. The
logistic regression analysis demonstrated that the best predictors of mortality, within six years of bereavement, were having no-one to telephone,

Table 1. LOGISTIC REGRESSION ANALYSIS OF FACTORS ASSOCIATED WITH MORTALITY AT SIX YEARS AFTER BEREAVEMENT

Variables associated with mortality at five years after bereavement	x2 value at six years after bereavement (controlling for age and sex as main effects)		
	Degrees freedom	x2 value	Significance level
No telephone contacts	1	5.7	0.02
Self reported nerves/ depression	1	5.0	0.05
Interviewer assessed depression	1	9.5	0.01
Interviewer assessed low happiness	2	6.8	0.05

self-reported and interviewer assessed problems with nerves and depression; and interviewer assessments of a low level of happiness, see Table 1.

Relative risk analysis showed that the widowed with these characteristics in 1979 had between almost two and three and a half times more chance of dying in the next six years (see Table 2). Although other measures of social support and contacts, emotional wellbeing and medication taking were also associated with increased risk of mortality, these did not reach statistical significance with the relative risk analysis. They should not be dismissed. The findings should be interpreted with some caution given the wide confidence intervals, due to small sample numbers. Because the sample was relatively small, it is possible that some real risk factors might not be found to be statistically significant. Attention should be given to the range of possible relative risks than merely to significant levels. Even when results were not statistically significant, the trends were in the expected direction, given the original hypotheses of the study (that a low level of social support and contact and poor emotional wellbeing would be associated with mortality after bereavement).

Table. 2. ESTIMATED RELATIVE RISKS OF MORTALITY FOR WIDOWS AND WIDOWERS UP TO SIX YEARS AFTER BEREAVEMENT*

Variables associated with increased risk+	Relative risk	95% confidence limit
Interviewer assessed depression	2.35	1.34 – 4.13
Interviwer assessment of low happiness level	3.41	1.29 – 9.05
No telephone contacts	1.98	1.12 – 3.50
Self reported nerves or depression	1.86	1.07 – 3.24

* All variables were dichotomised and risks are expressed relative to the alternative

+ Once adjusted for effects of age and sex by logistic regression

DISCUSSION

The implications of the statistical findings are that the best independent predictors of mortality were : poor emotional wellbeing on the basis of three of the emotional wellbeing measures and a single measure of social support : telephone contacts (telephone ownership was controlled for). It was found in 1979 that those with telephone contacts had the same social network size as others (in terms of numbers of relatives and friends, frequency seen, and availability of people they obtained comfort from etc.). It is possible that having someone to telephone may reflect a deeper level of psycho-social support than simply measuring frequency and type of social contacts. This may be particularly important for the elderly who may find it difficult to go out to visit relatives and friends, when company is needed, due to increasing frailty and possibly to lack of money and transport.

In 1979 it was found that those widowed who more often had difficulties accepting living alone, and who more often mentioned a relative or friend they would like to see (or see more often), were more likely to report problems with depression (Bowling and Cartwright, 1982). It has been hypothesised that social support can act as a buffer to feelings of emotional distress. These factors have been associated with physical and psychological health (Berkman and Syme, 1979). There is some evidence of the effects of the central nervous systems on immune function. It is thus possible that stress may have a biological effect partly through the immune system, the implication being that the immune system is engaged in the response to psychological stress (Anthony, 1987). It follows that the bereaved show increased morbidity and mortality, and reduced lymphocyte function has been documented following bereavement (Bartrop et al., 1977; Scheifer et al., 1983).

This study lends some support to the hypotheses that lower levels of social support and poorer emotional wellbeing are associated with a higher risk of mortality after bereavement. This is consistent with evidence from studies based on larger samples relating to the recorded cause of death among the recently widowed. Diseases of the heart and death from accidents, poisonings and violence are excessive among the widowed in comparison with the non-widowed of the same ages (Gove, 1973).

The general practitioner is the professional most likely to be in contact with the widowed, seeing three quarters of the widowed in this study in the early months of bereavement. The GP is therefore in a good position to assess their risk factors for mortality after bereavement, especially in relation to depression and social support. Cartwright (1982) has commented on the decline in home visiting among general practitioners. They are thus decreasingly likely to be fully aware of the home circumstances of their elderly and widowed patients. One of the recommendations of the 1979 study was that GPs should visit their elderly widowed patients at home in order to assess their circumstances. The follow up study of mortality after bereavement confirms the possible importance of this suggestion.

ACKNOWLEDGEMENTS

I would like to thank Dr Ann Cartwright for her continuous support and also Professor Bernard Benjamin and Mr John Charleton for their statistical help and advice. Thanks is also due to Anne Fleissig and Margaret Hall who coded and checked the data.

The survey of the widowed, and the flagging operation, was supported by the Department of Health and Social Security, Great Britain.

REFERENCES

Anthony, H., 1987, Measuring differences between individuals - medical measurements, Complementary Medical Research, 2:82-93.

Bartrop, R. W., Lazarus, L., Luckhurst, E., 1977, Depressed lymphocyte function after bereavement, Lancet, 1:834-836.

Berkman, L. F. and Syme, S. L., 1979, Social networks, host resistance and mortality : a nine year follow up study of Alameda county residents, American Journal of Epidemiology, 109:186-204.

Bloom, B. L., Asher, S. J. and White, S. W., 1978, Marital disruption as a stressor : a review and analysis, Psychology Bulletin, 85:867-894.

Bowling, A. and Cartwright, A., 1982, "Life after a Death. A Study of the Elderly Widowed", Tavistock Publications, London.

Bowling, A. and Benjamin, B., 1985, Mortality after bereavement. A follow up study of a sample of elderly widowed people, Biology and Society, 2:197-203.

Bowling, A., 1987, Mortality after bereavement: A review of the literature on survival periods and factors affecting survival, Social Science and Medicine, 24:117-124.

Carter, H. and Glick, P. C., 1976, "Marriage and Divorce: A Social and Economic Study" (rev.edn.), Harvard University Press, Cambridge, Mass.

Cartwright, A., 1982, The role of the general practitioner in helping the elderly widowed, Journal of the Royal College of General Practitioners, 32:215-227.

Gove, W. R., 1973, Sex, marital status and mortality, American Journal of Sociology, 79:49-67.

Gove, W. R. and Hughes, M., 1979, Possible causes of the apparent sex differences in physical health: an empirical investigation, American Sociological Review, 44:126-146.

Maddison, D. C. and Viola, A., 1968, The health of widows in the year following bereavement, Journal of Psychosomatic Research, 12:297-306.

Parkes, C. M. and Brown, R., 1972, Health after bereavement: a controlled study of young Boston widows and widowers, Psychosomatic Medicine, 34:449-461.

Parkes, C. M., 1975, Unexpected and untimely bereavement: a statistical study of young Boston widows and widowers, in "Bereavement: Its Psycho-social Aspects" (Edited by B. Schoenberg) Columbia University Press, New York.

Scheifer, S. J., Keller, S. E. and Camerino, M., 1983, Suppression of lymphocyte stimulation following bereavement, Journal of the American Association, 250:374-377.

ETHICAL IMPLICATIONS OF USE OF THE LIVING WILL IN

CARE OF THE TERMINALLY ILL

Robyn Shapiro

Medical College of Wisconsin
Milwaukee, U.S.A.

DEFINITION OF THE LIVING WILL

Medical technology now can sustain basic bodily functions long after active, conscious life is gone. However, not all terminally ill patients wish to take advantage of such technology; rather, some opt to die in a natural, dignified manner. The living will allows for this choice by declaring the signer's intent that no extraordinary means be used to prolong life should he or she suffer an illness or injury for which extraordinary care cannot provide a cure or effectuate significant recovery, and from which death is inevitable.

LEGAL SUPPORT FOR THE LIVING WILL

The notion of the living will is well grounded in American law. Both the doctrine of informed consent and one's constitutional right to privacy allow a terminal patient to refuse extraordinary medical treatment which will not provide cure or effectuate significant recovery. First, under informed consent, no medical procedure may be performed unless the patient agrees, after explanation of the nature of the treatment, the substantial risks, and alternative therapies. As explained by the Kansas Supreme Court:

"Anglo-American law starts with the premise of thoroughgoing self-determination. It follows that each man is considered to be master of his own body, and he may, if he be of sound mind, expressly prohibit the performance of life saving surgery or other medical treatment. A doctor might well believe that an operation or form of treatment is desirable or necessary, but the law does not permit him to substitute his own judgment for that of the patient by any form of artifice or deception." (1)

One's right to refuse treatment has also been upheld based on his constitutionally guaranteed right to privacy, which encompasses the right to refuse medical treatment. In In re Quinlan, 70 N.J. 10, 355 A.2d 647, cert. denied, 429 U.S. 922 (1976), involving a 20 year old woman in a permanently vegetative state whose guardian was allowed to discontinue her respirator; in Superintendent of Belchertown State School v. Saikewicz, 373 Mass. 728, 370 N.E.2d 417 (1977) where the court answered in the negative the question of whether Saikewicz, an incompetent 67 year old man, had to receive chemo-therapy treatments for incurable acute monocytic leukemia; (2) in Severns v.

Wilmington Medical Center, Inc., 421 A.2d 1334 (Del. Sup. Ct. 1980), granting the chancery court the power to allow the husband-guardian of an irreversibly comatose patient to order discontinuance of her respirator; in Satz v. Perlmutter, 379 So.2d 359 (Fla.1980), upholding discontinuance of a respirator for a 73 year old terminally ill man; and in In re Welfare of Colyer, 99 Wash. 2d. 114, 660 P. 2d 738 (1983), wherein life support systems for a woman in chronic vegetative state were discontinued, the courts' decisions were based on the patients' constitutional rights of privacy. (3)

In addition to this case-law support for the living will, 39 states in America, plus the District of Columbia, have passed statutes which explicitly authorize the execution of living wills. While these bills vary from state to state, living will legislation characteristicaly contains the following key provisions:

1. a requirement for medical confirmation of the patient's terminal condition;
2. a requirement that the document be made a part of its author's medical record;
3. immunity of physicians, other health practitioners, and health care facilities for complying with the patients instructions as outlined in the will;
4. censure of physicians for failure either to comply with the document or to transfer the patient to the care of another physician who will;
5. easy revocation procedures if the patient has a change of mind;
6. a form for the living will declaration;
7. procedures for executing the declaration;
8. a statement that execution of a will has no effect on the patient's life insurance or health care benefits.

PROBLEMS WITH LIVING WILL LEGISLATION

Some living will statutes contain restrictive provisions which hinder the utilization of such documents. For instance, Wisconsin's living will law, as originally passed, required 'terminal condition' before a living will could be honored, and it defined 'terminal condition' as that which 'reasonable medical judgment' concludes will result in death within 30 days. Two physicians were required to certify in writing that the patient would die within 30 days, regardless of whether life sustaining procedures were used. Given the difficulty of determining that death will occur within 30 days (as opposed to 31, 32 etc.), physicians understandably were reluctant to honor a living will, despite the legal liability protection section in the law; and it was in large part this reluctance which led to an amendment of that definition of 'terminal condition' in Wisconsin's law. (4)

Another controversial provision in Wisconsin's living will law is the exemption of the provision of fluid maintenance and nutritional support from the list of 'life sustaining procedures' which may be withdrawn or withheld. The law restrictively defines 'life sustaining procedures' which a living will declarant may refuse, as 'any medical procedure or intervention that, in the judgment of the attending physician, would serve only to prolong the dying process but not avert death when applied to a qualified patient'. 'Life sustaining procedures' include assistance in respiration, artificial maintenance of blood pressure and heart rate, blood transfusion, kidney dialysis, and other similar procedures. 'Life sustaining procedures' do not include the provision of fluid maintenance and nutritional support or the alleviation of pain by administering medication or by performing any medical procedure. Despite the legal liability protection section in the law, the express exclusion of 'nutritional support' from the definition of 'life sustaining procedures' may create great discomfort for the physician who, for example, feels that it would be medically inappropriate to provide hyperalimentation for the permanently vegetative, terminal cancer patient/ declarant who cannot be nutritionally supported any other way.

BENEFITS OF LIVING WILL LEGISLATION

Despite potential hinderance to living will utilization posed by controversial provisions in certain state laws, such as Wisconsin's, living will legislation is an important mechanism for protecting patient autonomy because it a) fosters communication between physician and patient regarding the patient's care at the end of life; and b) enhances the likelihood that living wills be honored by assuring legal protection for the physician who follows the terminally ill patient's non-treatment instructions.

(a) Fostering Physician/Patient Communication

Recent literature suggests that individual autonomy is restricted by widespread reluctance among physicians to discuss distressing prospects with their patients. In a recent study by Bedell and Delbanco about CPR (Cardio-pulmonary resuscitation) decision making, for instance, only 19% of the patients who were resuscitated had been asked earlier whether they wished cardiopulmonary resuscitation if it became necessary, despite the fact that 86% of the patients were competent and nearly all of the physicians favored participation of patients in these decisions "at least sometimes". (5) In almost the same number of cases, the families were consulted instead of the patients, although these patients were just as likely to be competent. According to Bedell and Delbanco, often the possibility of CPR was not dis-cussed because physicians felt that such discussion was unnecessary. The private physicians in particular ". . . believe(d) that the patients will initiate a discussion about resuscitation" if they wish to and that they will usually tell you in other ways besides words that they do (or do not) want to be resuscitated. In that survey, in 68% of the cases the physicians thought that they knew what the patients would have wished.

However, recent data indicate that physicians are wrong in their assumption that such discussion is unnecessary. Several surveys indicate that most people, whether well or seriously ill, wish to be informed of their condition and to participate in medical decisions. (6) And patient partici-pation via nonverbal communication is not accurate. Of the 24 competent patients in the Bedell/Delbanco study who survived to discharge, 8 stated that they had not desired CPR and would not want it again; yet only 1 of the 16 physicians caring for these 8 patients suspected that the patient felt this way. Furthermore, the wisdom of waiting for the patient to initiate the exchange of information necessary for joint decision making is question-able. The patient may not have information necessary to know when to speak and what is at stake, and he may be fearful that asking questions will offend the physician. The President's Commission for the Study of Ethical Problems in Medicine and Biomedical and Behavioral Research surveyed a large sample of the general public about who should initiate such conversations, and the results were as follows: 66% said that it is the doctor's responsibility to ensure that the patient is fully informed about his or her condition and treatment; 20% said that it is the patient's responsibility to ask; and 12% felt that they are equally responsible. (7)

The Bedell and Delbanco study indicated that in place of physician/ patient joint decision making, medical information and decisions are often shared with the competent patient's family. Even recent medical literature tacitly assumes the practice of consulting first with families. For example, the ninth edition of Harrison's Principles of Internal Medicine suggests that "the wishes of the family" be one determinant of "how much the patient is told". (8) Surveys of physicians show that 20% to 50% consider the family's wishes an important reason for withholding information from a patient. (9) This implies that many physicians talk first with the family; and, depending upon the outcome of that conversation, they may not discuss substantive issues with the patient at all. Without information, the patient cannot participate in decisions.

Living will legislation may foster more open and meaningful dialogue between physicians and patients on issues surrounding terminal care. Indeed, in a survey of Wisconsin physicians regarding their knowledge of and attitudes towards the state's Living Will law, nearly 50% of the respondents said that the legislation would be helpful in their practice in terms of clarifying patients' wishes, making such decisions easier, and supporting the practice of humane medicine. (10)

(b) Protecting Physician Compliance with Living Wills

Even in the absence of living will statutes, living wills are legally binding by the force of case law protecting one's right to refuse medical treatment. Despite such case law support, however, physicians fear criminal and/or civil legal liability for following living will directives. Some, for instance, fear that homicide charges will be brought if they discontinue life prolonging treatment for a terminally ill patient pursuant to his living will. Some fear civil malpractice liability if they appropriately honor a living will. Living will statutes legislatively affirm that physicians who comply with living wills will not be civilly or criminally liable; and in so clarifying such legal protection, the legislative intent, most likely, was to promote utilization of living wills. Indeed, the physicians surveyed in the Wisconsin study overwhelmingly (more than 94%) supported the provision in Wisconsin's law which relieves them from civil or criminal liability and charges of unprofessional conduct for actions taken in accordance with the declaration's provisions. (11)

The importance of living will legislation, which promotes the utilization of advance directives, becomes all the more clear in comparison to medical treatment decision making for incompetent terminal patients who have not executed advance directives. Until very recently, the only way to insure that reliance on family consent to withdraw or withhold treatment would not subject a health care provider to the risk of civil or criminal liability was to go to court, either to have a family member appointed by a court as the patient's legal guardian or to obtain judicial approval of the decision itself. Going to court, however, can be humiliating for the patient and family and expensive in terms of resources and time. Fortunately, in recent years, courts in 5 different states (Arizona(12), California(13), Connecticut(14), Florida(15), and Washington(16)) have authorised the families of adult patients to exercise the right of the patient to forego treatment without going to court; in Massachusetts, courts have upheld the validity of do not resuscitate orders approved by family members(17); and legislatures in 11 states (Arkansas, Connecticut, Florida, Iowa, Louisiana, New Mexico, North Carolina, Oregon, Texas, Utah, and Virginia) have passed statutes authorizing families to exercise the right of specified patients to stop or forego life prolonging treatment. (18) To the extent reliance on families means faster and less expensive decision making with no diminution in the quality of the decision made, this trend should be welcomed.

However, the trend towards reliance on families is not without problems. First the term "family" is not very precise. When relatives disagree as to what the patient would want, therefore, the dispute will probably require court resolution, at least in the absence of law which specifies whose decision is to be given priority. In addition, the family may not include the most knowledgeable proxy decision maker. Thus, even if a patient has lived for years with someone who is not a relative, the non-relative will have authority to speak for the patient only if he is designated as the proxy by the patient in an advance directive. A more serious problem with reliance on family consent to withhold treatment is how to protect patients from families who decide on the basis of ignorance or in bad faith. While there should be a legal presumption in favor of family consent, in some cases that presumption must be challenged, for good reason, by an ethics committee or through judicial review. In this regard, physicians are likely to be uncomfortable with the responsibility of assessing whether family members are acting in good faith.

The living will is not only preferable to reliance on family consent for medical treatment withdrawal from incompetent terminal patients; it is preferable to utilization of durable powers of attorney. All states in America have durable power of attorney statutes which permit individuals to delegate to another the legal authority to act on their behalf after they become incapacitated. Enacted primarily with property matters in mind (e.g. to authorize the writing of checks on the principal's behalf), most durable power of attorney statutes are silent about health care matters. However, some statutes do address health care decision making; and attorneys believe that even in the others, the authority may be applied to medical treatment decisions if the principal has so specified.

There are several drawbacks to utilization of the durable power of attorney for health care decision making. First, this method of controlling terminal treatment is limited by the reality that many people, especially among the elderly, have no one to appoint. Second, even if an agent has been appointed under a durable power of attorney statute, the agent may not be available when a treatment decision needs to be made; or (s)he may have a conflict of interest, either emotionally or legally.

CONCLUSION

Utilization of the living will avoids legal uncertainties of family consent, and, in many states, of utilization of durable power of attorney for treatment decision making; it avoids the possibility of ignorant or ill-founded decisions by proxies; and it alleviates the burden that being a proxy decision maker places on loved ones. To the extent that one's living will cannot predict all the various alternatives that become possible as acute illnesses arise, perhaps it should include a clause directing that a certain individual be contacted for interpretation of the document, should that be necessary. Greater use of such living will directives should be encouraged to more effectively and efficiently promote good medical decision making and protection of patient autonomy.

REFERENCES

1. Natanson v. Kline, 186 Kansas Supreme Court 393, 406–07, 350 P.2d 1093, 1104 (1960).
2. In Superintendent of Belchertown State School v. Saikewicz, 373 Mass. 728, 742, 370 N.E.2d 417, 426 (1977) the court described: "The constitutional right to privacy, as we conceive it, is an expression of the sanctity of individual free choice and self-determination as fundamental constituents of life. The value of life as so perceived is lessened not by a decision to refuse treatment, but by the failure to allow a competent human being the right of choice."
3. Many lower state courts have also cited the right to privacy in upholding the patient's right to refuse medical treatment. See, e.g. Leach v. Akron General Medical Center, 58 Ohio Misc 1, 426 N.E.2d 809

(C.P. Summit Co. P. Div. 1980), where the court granted the guardian of a terminally ill, permanently vegetative woman the power to direct discontinuance of her respirator, based on her constitutional right to privacy.

4. Wisconsin's living will law, as amended, defines "terminal condition" as "an incurable condition caused by injury or illness that reasonable medical judgement finds would cause death imminently, so that the application of life-sustaining procedures serves only to postpone the moment of death."

5. S.E. Bedell and T.L. Delbanco, Choices About Cardiopulmonary Resuscitation in the Hospital: When do Physicians Talk with Patients? N. Eng. J. Med. 310:1089-93 (1984).

6. See President's Commission for the Study of Ethical Problems in Medicine and Biomedical and Behavioral Research. "Summing Up", Washington, D.C. Government Printing Office, 1983; R.M. Veatch, "Death, Dying and the Biological Revolution: Our Last Quest for Responsibility", New Haven, Conn: Yale University press, 204-48 (1976); N.H. Cassem and R.S. Stewart, Management and Care of the Dying Patient, Int. J. Psychiatry Med. 6:293-304 (1975).

7. President's Commission for the Study of Ethical Problems in Medicine and Biomedical and Behavioral Research, "Making Health Care Decisions", Vol. 2., Washington, D.C. : Government Printing Office, 116 (1982).

8. K.J. Isselbacher, R.D. Adams, E. Braunwald, R.G. Petersdorf and J.D. Wilson, eds., "Harrison's Principles of Internal Medicine", 9th ed., McGraw-Hill, New York, 6 (1980).

9. D.H. Novack, R. Plumer, R.L. Smith, H. Ochitill, G.R. Morrow and J.M. Bennett, "Changes in Physicians' Attitudes Towards Telling the Cancer Patient", JAMA, 241:897-900 (1979); Presidents Commission for the Study of Ethical Problems in Medicine and Biomedical and Behavioral Research "Making Health Care Decisions" Vol. 2, Washington D.C., Government Printing Office, 145 (1982).

10. R. Shapiro, "Living Will in Wisconsin", Wisconsin Medical Journal Vol.85 17-23 (1986).

11. Ibid.

12. Rasmussen v. Fleming, No. 2 CA-CIV 5622 (Ariz Ct App, June 25, 1986).

13. Barber v. Superior Court, 147 Cal App 3d 1006, 195 Cal Rptr 484 (1983).

14. Foody v. Manchester Memorial Hospital, 40 Conn. Super. 127, 482 A 2d 713 (Conn. Super. Ct. 1984).

15. John F. Kennedy Hospital v. Bludworth, 452 So. 2d 921 (Fla. 1984).

16. In re Colyer, 99 Wash. 2d 114, 660 P 2d 738 (1983) (en banc).

17. In re Dinnerstein, 6 Mass app 629, 405 NE 2d 115 (1980).

18. See Ark Stat Ann Sec 82-3803; Conn Gen Stat Ann Sec. 19a-571; Fla Stat Ch 84-58 sec. 765.07; Iowa Code ch 144A.7; La Rev. Stat. 40:1299.58.5; NM Stat Ann Sec. 24-7-8.1; NC Gen Stat Sec. 90-322; Or Rev. Stat. Sec. 97.083; Tex Stat Ann Art 4590h, Sec. 4C; Utah Code Ann Sec. 75-2-1107; Va Code Sec. 54-325.8:6.

PART TWO

VARIETIES OF CARING RESPONSES

PAIN TREATMENT AND TERMINAL CARE IN FINNISH HOSPITALS

Anneli Vainio

Helsinki University Central Hospital
Helsinki, Finland

In Finland, with a population of about 5 million, the number of patients dying of malignant diseases is 10,000 a year. Almost all of them (93%) die in hospitals, 2% in other institutions, and only 5% die at home. During the last few years, increasing attention has been paid to the quality of terminal care. New ideas about individual and comprehensive care have entered into the Finnish communal home care system, and the first hospice is under construction.

The National Board of Health in Finland published its instructions for terminal care in 1982, emphasizing the humane qualities of the care. According to the instructions, terminal care should aim to give the patient a possibility to live his last days without pain and other distressing symptoms, in a surrounding which he can choose himself, with his beloved persons around him. The care-giving personnel should have sufficient know-ledge, skills and a positive attitude toward the proper realization of terminal care. Special attention should be paid to the relief of pain.

The instructions offer a challenge to the personnel working with the terminal ill. How does the health care system meet the demands of skills and compassion? A recent questionnaire survey, where 783 Finnish physicians were interviewed, revealed a severe undertreatment of the pain of terminal cancer patients (Vainio). About half of the physicians failed to treat the pain effectively in three simulated patient examples. Weak anti-inflammatory analgesics were suggested for severe cancer pain, and in cases where narcotic analgesics were recommended, most daily doses represented 30-60% of the minimal analgesic doses of the drugs. No studies are available on the quality of terminal care in Finland, in contrast to countries with a network of hospices, where the tradition of the self-assessment of care is well developed.

The aims of this study are: (i) to obtain an overall view of the prevalence of pain among dying cancer patients, (ii) to evaluate the quality of pain treatment and (iii) to assess the adequacy of psychological support in Finnish hospitals, as it is experienced by the closest relatives of the patients. The bereaved family members' suggestions about how hospitals could better help dying patients will be presented as well.

METHODS

A questionnaire was sent to the closest relatives, as defined by the hospital routine, of 550 cancer patients, who died in seven Finnish hospitals in 1984. The hospitals were selected to represent different levels of the Finnish health care system and different parts of the country. There were two clinics of a university hospital, (surgery, 43 patients, and oncology, 176 patients), one central hospital (175), two district hospitals (125) and two small local hospitals (31 patients), situated in rural and urban areas. The names and addresses of the nearest relatives were obtained from the patients' case records, which were selected by diagnosis from the hospitals' yearly statistics. The questionnaires were sent 6-12 months after the death of the patients.

The questionnaire consisted of 21 multiple-choice questions. After the questions, the respondents were asked to freely express their comments and suggestions regarding the care of a dying patient in a hospital. The comments were categorized by analyzing the subsample of the 50 first answers.

The intensity of pain was evaluated with a 4-step verbal scale (agonizing-severe-moderate-mild). The treatment of pain was scaled similarly (good-fair-insufficient-poor). In questions concerning psychological support to the patient and to the respondent himself, the amount of support was evaluated dichotomously (enough/not enough). In every question, the possibility of not having an opinion/not knowing was also given.

To obtain background information for the fairly simple scaling of pain treatment (good-fair-insufficient-poor), the family members' opinions of pain treatment were analyzed separately in subgroups of different pain intensity and continuity, psychological support by physicians, and of respondents who expressed spontaneous complaints about pain treatment or about physicians.

RESULTS

Of the closest relatives of 550 cancer patients, 27 were not reached, and the letters were returned by the post. Nineteen relatives returned the questionnaires unanswered for the following reasons: Eleven relatives were dead. Three did not understand Finnish, two did not want to answer because they were disappointed in the health care system, and three were too ill to answer. Eighty-four relatives did not return the questionnaires. Four hundred and twenty questionnaires (76%) were analyzed.

The mean age of the respondents was 54 years (range 17-86). Fifty-five percent were spouses, 5% parents, 27% children, 6% sisters and brothers, 5% other relatives, and 2% friends of the deceased patients. Seventy-three percent had visited the hospital daily, 22% at least once a week, and 5% at longer intervals. The distance to the hospital varied from 1 to 800 km, being less than 10 km in 53%. The patient's last stay in the hospital varied from one day to two years, the mean being 45 days.

The prevalence of pain was 74%, as reported by the relatives. The intensity of pain was estimated as agonizing in 22%, severe in 44%, moderate in 20% and mild in 7%. Seven percent of the respondents were not aware of the intensity of pain. One third of the patients had had continuous pain, two thirds intermittent pain. The duration of pain had been several years in 30%, several months in 60%, and weeks in 10%.

Less than half of the respondents found that the patients had got enough psychological support from the hospital staff (Table 1). Both the patients

Table 1. PSYCHOLOGICAL SUPPORT GIVEN BY THE HOSPITAL STAFF TO THE PATIENT AND TO THE FAMILY MEMBERS AS EVALUATED BY THE FAMILY MEMBER (N=420)

	Satisfactory %	Unsatisfactory %	Cannot Say %
Support to the patient			
Physician	31	26	43
Nurses	46	19	35
Hospital priest	16	11	73
Social worker	20	13	67
Support to the family member			
Physician	34	44	22
Nurses	44	32	24

and the family members got less psychological support from the physicans than from the nurses. Fourteen percent of the respondents had met the hospital priest, and 20% had met the social worker. When visiting the hospital, 79% of the respondents felt that the attitude of the personnel towards them had been friendly. Seven percent felt it was hostile or indifferent, and for 11% it was sometimes friendly, sometimes cold. Three percent did not know. Between the different types of hospitals, there were no systematic differences in the evaluation of psychological support.

The majority of the respondents (64%) thought that the presence of trained volunteers in the hospital wards could benefit the dying patients. Negative were 6%, and 30% had no opinion. A majority of the family members (61%) would also have been willing to meet a member of the hospital staff after the death of the patient, had it been possible. 21% were not willing, and 18% had no opinion. For 56%, the best time would have been a week after the death, 28% preferred a month, and 16% several months.

When asked, what would have been the best place to die for their family member, 21% preferred home (Table 2). A hospital near home (a local hospital) was appreciated by 39%, and a specialist clinic (university or central hospital) by 33% of the respondents. Other institutions were suggested by three percent, and four percent had no opinion. For the majority of the respondents who preferred a hospital, the type of hospital corresponded to the institution where their family member had actually been treated.

The relatives were also asked about the kind of help that would have been necessary, if they had cared for their dying family member at home. Half of the respondents would have needed nursing help. Cleaning-up services, substitutes for family members when going out, catering and laundry services would have been necessary as well, mentioned in this order.

After the multiple-choice questions, the family members were asked to

Table 2. THE DESIRED PLACE OF TERMINAL CARE BY THE ACTUAL PLACE OF
DYING, AS EXPRESSED BY THE FAMILY MEMBERS

	Actual place of treatment				
Desired place of treatment	University hospital N=162 %	Central hospital N=115 %	District hospital N=103 %	Local hospital N=27 %	Total N=407 %
Home	22	14	29	12	21
University or central hospital	51	32	15	7	33
District or local hospital	24	47	47	70	39
Other	2	3	5	0	3
No opinion	1	4	4	11	4
	100	100	100	100	100

freely express their comments or suggestions regarding the care of a dying
patient in the hospital. Two hundred and ninety-five comments were written,
analyzed in Table 3. A majority of the comments contained critical remarks
about everyday hospital practice as well as about the work and behaviour of
the staff. In the table, the comments are categorized according to the
objects. When picking out the most frequent complaints of each object, the
dying patient's loneliness in hospital becomes stressed as the principal
problem. This topic was expressed in 121 comments complaining that the
physicians and nurses had too little time for the patients, were difficult to
reach when needed, or were too few. Better possibilities for the family
members to stay with the dying patient were wished as well, as illustrated
by the following citations: "The patient was often left alone for hours,
isolated (infection) and with difficulties to breathe. The nursing care was
superficial, and the family members often had to ask for help and alleviation." "The physician had never time to discuss about my mother." "Even
a telephone call was too much for the busy doctors." "Everything happened so
quickly. I spent the morning in the corridor. I wanted to stay with my
mother, but I was let in for only a couple of minutes before she died."

The lack of information to the family about the patient's situation was
seen as a problem as well, being the subject of 39 comments. "I was not told
that it was cancer. Two days before my husband's death I was told that he
may die at any time. This was a total surprise to me."

About ten percent of the comments dealt with poor pain treatment, and
the tone of the complaints expressed a deep concern of the subject. "I had
to remind constantly about the pain medication. The nurses seemed indifferent. My mother trembled with pain every time the previous medication wore

Table 3. THE FAMILY MEMBER'S COMMENTS ABOUT TERMINAL CARE IN HOSPITAL

		Number of comments	%
Complaints of negligence in symptom relief		40	14
Pain	30		
Other symptoms	10		
Comments about physicians		56	19
Difficult to reach	24		
Too little time for patient	16		
Abrupt behaviour	10		
Changing too often	6		
Comments about nurses		62	21
Should have more time to stay with the patient	38		
Abrupt behaviour	13		
Rough handling of the patients	5		
Negligence in patient care	6		
Comments about hospital practice and organisation		59	20
Family should be allowed to stay longer with the patient	24		
Too few nurses	19		
Language problems	6		
Physical isolation/dreary surroundings	6		
Difficulties in admission	4		
Comments about information to the relatives		39	13
The family should be told more explicitly about the approaching death	21		
More precise information about the diagnosis needed	15		
The information was given in a too harsh manner	3		
Thanks and positive comments		22	7
Friendly hospital staff	11		
Good nursing care	7		
Good medical care	4		
Other comments		17	6
		295	100

Table 4. THE FAMILY MEMBERS' OPINION ABOUT PAIN TREATMENT BY THE INTENSITY AND CONTINUITY OF PAIN

Pain treatment evaluated by family member	The intensity and persistence of pain reported			
	Agonizing or severe	Moderate or mild	Continuous	Intermittent
	N=237 %	N=95 %	N=97 %	N=230 %
Good	45	43	41	48
Fair	43	40	43	40
Insufficient	6	1	6	4
Cannot say	6	16	10	8
Total	100	100	100	100

Table 5. THE FAMILY MEMBERS' OPINION ABOUT PAIN TREATMENT BY THE PSYCHOLOGICAL SUPPORT GIVEN BY PHYSICIANS, AND THEIR SPONTANEOUS COMPLAINTS ABOUT PHYSICIANS

Pain treatment evaluated by family member	Sufficient psychological support by physician	Insufficient psychological support by physician	Complaints about physicians
	N=111 %	N=99 %	N=52 %
Good	65	24	32
Fair	28	60	52
Insufficient	2	11	8
Cannot say	5	5	8
Total	100	100	100

off. This happened in spite of the physician's direction." "The patient had excruciating pain. The tests were not yet completed, therefore no medication was given. There was the physician and a nurse. He died on the same day."

When asked specifically, the treatment of pain was evaluated by the family members as good in 45%, fair in 41% and insufficient or poor in 4%. A tenth of the respondents could not evaluate the treatment. The type of hospital had no significant effect on the evaluation of pain treatment. In Tables 4-5, the opinions of pain treatment are analyzed by several other parameters. The intensity or continuity of the patient's pain had no effect on the opinion about pain treatment. The respondents, who either expressed complaints about the behaviour of physicians, or reported that the patient received no physical support from them, were less satisfied with the pain treatment, too. Eighteen (62%) of the 30 respondents who spontaneously complained about poor pain treatment, reported it as good or fair when it was asked directly. Eight (28%) of these respondents evaluated it as insufficient.

DISCUSSION

The aim of this study was to get an overall view of the quality of terminal care in Finnish hospitals. Seven hospitals in different parts of the country were therefore chosen. For this geographic reason, it was not possible to conduct personal interviews of the patients, and the physical and psychological fragility of terminal cancer patients prevented the use of questionnaires. Because doctors and nurses working at hospitals are part of the system, they were thought to be biased in its favour.

C.M. Parkes (1978-1985) successfully used the interview of surviving spouses in the comparative evaluations of terminal care at home, hospital and hospice. Hinton (1979) interviewed terminal cancer patients, their spouses and nurses about the quality of care in different settings. The ratings of these groups showed agreement with correlations of about 0.6. Morris et al.(1986) compared the evaluation of pain by patients and their primary care persons. The correlation of the reports was 0.43. Thus, the family members of patients can be regarded as a relatively reliable source of information. In the present study, the reliability of the information from the closest family members is enhanced by the fact that 73% of them visited the hospital daily.

Because many of the respondents were thought to be old and in poor condition, the questions were formulated as simple as possible. The relatively high response rate of 77% indicates that the questions were not too difficult, and that the respondents felt it important to answer. This was confirmed by 50 letters to the author, spontaneously enclosed with the questionnaires.

The family members' judgements about hospital care may have been distorted by idealization and the need to believe that everything was done to help the patient. Conversely, the bitterness and resentment which are common features of grief may well have made some of the family members excessively critical. By sending questionnaires 6-12 months after the patients' death it was hoped to eliminate some of the bias. However, the questionnaires seemed to re-evoke painful feelings connected with the loss of the dear person, as reported spontaneously by many respondents.

The family members' reports about the presence of pain in terminal cancer patients, 74%, is consistent with earlier reports on the subject. In the calculations of Bonica (1985) comprising data on 7700 patients, the prevalence of terminal pain was 71%.

The treatment of pain was judged to be good or fair in the majority of cases. This is a surprising finding, because numerous investigations about the quality of pain treatment in terminal cancer in different countries including Finland, indicate severe undertreatment.

The formulation of the question "Do you consider the pain treatment of your family member good/fair/insufficient/poor?" might be one reason for this finding. The evaluation of the respondent in this particular case depends on his expectations and the concept of what is good pain treatment. Levin and Cleeland (1985) examined public attitudes towards cancer pain by interviewing 496 persons by telephone. Their study revealed that cancer and pain are strongly linked in the public view; 57% of the respondents thought that cancer patients usually die a painful death. It is possible that the people in the present study were not aware that cancer pain can be relieved, and they did not expect their family members to be pain-free when on analgesic medication. This is supported by the fact that also 20 of the 30 respondents who complained about unrelieved pain in their free comments, judged the pain treatment as good or fair when asked directly (Table 5).

Another interesting fact is that the intensity of the patient's pain had no influence on the evaluation of pain treatment (Table 4). The judgements were similar in cases of agonizing/severe and moderate/mild pain. The same is reported in the study by Daut and Cleeland (1982), where there was no correlation between the percentage of relief reported by patients and the severity of their pain ratings.

The results of this study reflect the experiences of a random sample of the population, who became involved with the hospital through the fatal illness of their family member. It also describes the needs and expectations of cancer patients and their families, concerning the terminal care in hospital. Some general statements can be made about the adequacy of the care in the present system.

1) The dying patient is left too much alone in a hospital. In the present situation, there are no resources to provide dying patients with care-giving persons for a longer time than is required for routine physical and medical assistance. In many cases, the hospital routine also prevents the family members from staying long enough with the patients. The majority of family members would not object against trained volunteers. The family members could take care of dying people at home more than at present, provided that nursing help were available when needed.

2) The patients and their families do not get the psychological support and understanding that they need in this situation. The support should extend also to the period after the death in form of contacts between the family and the personnel of the hospital ward. In problematic cases, trained psychologists or family therapeutics should be available to assist the personnel.

3) The physicians' and nurses' skills in goal-directed symptom control, especially in pain relief, are still insufficient, and to some extent also neglected.

It should be recognized that dying patients in hospitals have different needs than those who are going to be cured. In terminal care, an orientation from the administration-centred way of thinking towards a more individually oriented way is necessary. One of the respondents of this questionnaire study expressed himself: "I wish there were a hospital where the routine and regulations were not the most important things, and where there would be a little bit of warmth and consideration of feelings".

ACKNOWLEDGEMENT

I wish to sincerely thank Elina Hemminki, Assistant Professor in Public Health, for her helpful advice in planning the questionnaire and for reviewing the paper.

REFERENCES

Bonica, J. J., 1985, Treatment of cancer pain. Current status and future needs, in: "Advances in Pain Research and Therapy", H.L. Fields, ed., Raven Press, New York.

Daut, R. L. and Cleeland, C. S., 1982, Prevalence and severity of pain in cancer, Cancer, 50:1913.

Hinton, J., 1979, Comparison of places and policies for terminal care, The Lancet, Jan 6:29.

Levin, D. N. and Cleeland, C. S., 1985, Dar R. Public attitudes toward Cancer Pain, Cancer, 56:2337.

Morris, J. N., Mor, V., Goldberg, R. J., Sherwood, S., Greer, D. S., Hiris, J., 1986, The effect of treatment setting and patient characteristics on pain in terminal cancer patients: a report from the National Hospice Study, J. Chron. Dis, 39:27.

Parkes, C. M., 1978, Home or hospital? Terminal care as seen by surviving spouses, Journal of the Royal College of General Practitioners 28:19.

Parkes, C. M. 1979, Terminal care: evaluation of in-patient service at St Christopher's Hospice Part I. Views of surviving spouse on effects of the service on the patient, Postgraduate Medical Journal, 55:517.

Parkes, C. M. 1979, Terminal care: evaluation of in-patient service at St Christopher's Hospice Part II, Self-assessments of effects of the service on surviving spouses, Postgraduate Medical Journal, 55:523.

Parkes, C. M., 1980, Terminal care: evaluation of an advisory domiciliary service at St Christopher's Hospice, Postgraduate Medical Journal, 56:685.

Parkes, C. M., 1984, 'Hospice' versus 'hospital' care - re-evaluation after 10 years as seen by surviving spouses, Postgraduate Medical Journal, 60:120.

Parkes, C. M., 1985, Terminal care: Home hospital or hospice?, The Lancet. Jan 19:155.

SPECIAL EQUIPMENT* FOR THE SEVERELY DISABLED

Richard Schilling and Peter Millard

Possum Controls
London, U.K.

INTRODUCTION

A challenge facing hospice and geriatric teams is to give their patients the 'fullest potential for living' before death (Saunders, 1986). While their priorities are to relieve pain, provide physical and spiritual comfort, an important aspect of their task is to maintain the dignity and self respect of people in their care. Dependent patients, constrained by illness and disability, with no means of contributing to life, become apathetic and depressed. The provision of equipment which affords them some control of their environment, improves the quality of life and helps to dispel apathy and depression (Millard and Smith, 1981).

There are three distinct groups of special equipment for the severely disabled which assist in providing mobility, environmental control and communication.

HELPING MOBILITY

The provision of equipment to help mobility is not within the remit of Possum Controls but it is important that aids to mobility such as walking sticks, zimmer frames and wheelchairs are not forgotten.

Electric wheelchairs should be considered. Even in the terminal stages of a non-dementing illness, the disabled sick can reach new goals.

Encouraging freedom to move within the confines of a ward from the dayroom to the bedside can transform the life of a handicapped person and give an element of choice.

PROVIDING ENVIRONMENTAL CONTROLS

Control of the environment depends on the ability to switch lights on and off, adjust the temperature, draw curtains, answer and make telephone

---

* Provided by Possum Controls Ltd., which is a charity owned organization dedicated to the development and production of a wide range of equipment to help the physically and mentally handicapped, the deaf and the blind. Profits are devoted to research and the provision of back-up services.

calls and open and close doors. Resiting switches or replacing them with alternative types of switch may be all that is necessary to give persons confined to wheelchairs the ability to control their environment.

The provision of environmental equipment can bring such control within a disabled person's capabilities, by means of sophisticated switch systems worked manually, by foot or head, by sucking and blowing or other inputs depending upon the degree of disability. Switches can be grouped together and placed within the disabled person's reach; for example, the Possum Link (PSU2) has a panel of six simple flick controls for an alarm, intercom, doorlock and three appliances.

If disability is so severe that movement is minimal or uncontrolled, a selector system is used. The Possum PSU3 is a Selector Unit operated by a single movement, eg. sucking or blowing through a mouthpiece or light finger pressure on a microswitch. This starts a selector 'stepping' through a number of switch control positions: when reached the equipment is switched on or off. Illuminated display panels indicate the on or off state of each appliance and contain an audible tone to assist the blind or partially sighted. In addition to the usual environmental controls, the PSU3 can be used to operate page-turners, select television and radio channels and operate a cassette tape recorder.

IMPROVING COMMUNICATIONS

Many elderly disabled and terminal care patients who have difficulties in speaking, writing and hearing, can be helped by slow clear speaking of staff and relatives and other means appropriate to their problems. Possum Controls produce portable communicators, such as the Porta-scan. This is ideal for carrying on the lap tray of a wheelchair. It can be operated by the built-in plate switch.

Special communication aids, however, are necessary for patients with motor neurone disease and cerebral palsy, who cannot speak or write, and in conditions such as multiple sclerosis and Huntington's chorea – where the patient can speak but cannot write. Possum have developed systems whereby a very disabled person can use a modified electric typewriter for written communication, often in conjunction with the PSU3. And like the PSU3, it is operated by a microswitch or gentle puffing and sucking on a tube. Letters are selected by a scanning light on an indicator panel. Text processors can be added to the system to allow compositions to be changed prior to typing or stored for future use. Typewriters can be operated through a special kind of expanded keyboard, designed for those with gross uncontrolled movements, such as sufferers from Huntington's chorea, multiple sclerosis and cerebral palsy. There is a mini keyboard system for those with limited hand movements, eg. in muscular dystrophy and osteopetrosis.

A newly designed electronic system which combines the functions of the PSU3 and the typewriter will be available in 1988, making communication and environmental control much easier.

SUPPLY OF EQUIPMENT THROUGH GOVERNMENT HEALTH DEPARTMENTS

Some 2,000 of the 150,000 severely handicapped in the United Kingdom are provided free of charge with the PSU3 environmental control system or typewriters for communication, which are fully maintained and serviced through the Department of Health and Social Security in England, the Welsh Office in Wales, and the Scottish Home and Health Department in Scotland and the Eastern Health and Social Services Board in Northern Ireland. They have to meet the criteria of disability set out by these Health Departments (DHSS 1983).

For an environmental control system, patients have to be so paralysed or so disabled by disease, injury or congenital defect that they are unable to carry out simple tasks in their homes. Another condition is that, without the apparatus, they would not be able to derive some continuing measure of independence and could not be assisted so effectively by simpler or cheaper means.

Where the speech of a severely disabled person, who is eligible for an environmental control system, is no longer intelligible and he or she is otherwise unable to communicate satisfactorily, a communication aid (Typewriter) may also be provided. In exceptional cases where full-time nursing or parental care is provided, the communication aid may be supplied on its own but eligibility for an environmental control system must be demonstrated.

FURTHER MEANS OF OBTAINING EQUIPMENT

Other units like pendant alarms, page-turners and portable communicators are not provided through Government Health Departments. They are frequently supplied by Social Services Departments and charitable organizations, which deal with special disabilities.

The Possum Trust, a registered charity, helps to supply equipment to those who cannot get funding from other sources.

PATIENTS CURRENTLY USING POSSUM EQUIPMENT

The most frequent types of disability in those using the PSU3 are multiple sclerosis (40%), motor neurone disease (13%), spinal injury (13%), cerebral palsy (12%) and rheumatoid arthritis (5%). Rarer groups include syringomyelia, muscular dystrophy, myasthenia gravis, Friedrich's ataxia and cerebral haemorrhage (stroke). An analysis of patients using typewriters (usually with the PSU3) shows that cerebral palsy (65%) is the most frequent type of disability; followed by multiple sclerosis (15%), motor neurone disease (8%) and other progressive neurological disorders and very rarely cerebral haemorrhage (stroke) and osteopetrosis.

An analysis of the users of Possum equipment reveals that very few are elderly (Table 1). In a sample supplied with the PSU3 Environmental Control System, 8% were over the age of 65. Two percent in this older group had been supplied with an electric typewriter; yet as many as 75% of the severely disabled in the United Kingdom are over 65 years old (Harris et al. 1971).

Table 1

Age Distribution of 178 patients using Possum Equipment

Age (yrs)	(1) PSU3	(2) Typewriter	(1)+(2)	Percent
< 25	19	46	65	(36.5)
25-64	67	36	103	(57.9)
65+	8	2	10	(5.6)
	94	84	178	(100.0)

Table 2

Table 2

Types of Terminal illnesses other than Cancer admitted by Hospices and Home
Care Teams

      motor neurone disease   Parkinsons's disease
      multiple sclerosis   rheumatoid and chr. arthritis
      Huntington's chorea   severe stroke
      muscular dystrophy   obstructive airways disease

Potential Value in Terminal Care

Hospices are concerned mainly with caring for patients with terminal
cancer, for whom this type of equipment has a limited value. However, a
survey undertaken by the St Christopher's Hospice Information Service in
1986 reveals that 51 out of the 121 Inpatient Units in the U.K. admitted, or
would consider admitting, patients with terminal illnesses other than cancer.
Nineteen Home Care teams and 5 Hospital-based Support teams gave a similar
reply.

Some Units were prepared to admit any patient in need of terminal care,
either respite or long term. Almost all specified the nature of the illness
which included most of those for which Possum equipment can help the sufferer
(Table 2). Motor Neurone disease (MND) was mentioned by almost every Unit;
other progressive neurological disorders were accepted by about half the
Units.

MND is a relatively rare disorder with a prevalence of 5 per 100,000
(Oliver et al, 1986). Because of the severe disability it causes, particularly dysarthria which occurs in about 75% of patients and its relatively
low mean duration of survival (3 years), hospices are able to provide the
special care which MND sufferers need. Patients may be loath to accept
these equipment aids because it is felt that they are a sign of deterioration.
Nevertheless, once accepted, they can be used for environmental control as
well as communication.

In the words of a patient (Ted Holden, 1980) with advanced MND, "I
have Possum equipment which gives me control of radio, television and the
typewriter. The typewriter is a great boon. Apart from the obvious aid in
communication, which is invaluable, it demands great concentration and
application and is, therefore, positive ......".

Both the typewriter and the PSU3 are being increasingly used by MND
sufferers. During the first 3 months of 1987, out of 64 patients, newly
supplied with these devices, 14 (22%) had MND compared with a corresponding
figure of 5%, 10 years ago.

Supplying Equipment

Providers of care, nurses, therapists and physicians should identify
patients needing this kind of equipment because it will help the terminally
ill to make a positive contribution to life and relieve some of the pressure
on nursing staff. In addition, hospice staff in collaboration with designers
and producers, can further the development of equipment aids for the severely
handicapped. Urgent action is needed. A recent survey funded by the Trent
Regional Health Authority (Wilkes, 1984), revealed a poor, and in some cases
a very poor, quality of life in 44% of terminally ill patients and a need for
more equipment.

Awareness that the terminally ill, in many cases, need equipment without delay, is paramount. The usual procedure whereby approval has to be

given by the Regional Assessor from the Health Department as to eligibility and type of system to be provided is inappropriate. There must be other means of supply; for example a pool, at a regional point, of PSU3s and type-writers which would be readily available. The assessment could be either by a member of the hospice staff who has been trained to do this type of work or by Possum. A possible option would be to have environmentally controlled bedrooms permanently set up in hospices.

Conclusion

Some 2,000 severely handicapped people in the United Kingdom are supplied free of charge by Government Health Departments with Environmental Control and typewriter systems which are fully maintained and serviced. Bearing in mind their types of disability, this equipment should be of value to patients in terminal care and, therefore, more widely used in hospices, special homes and departments of geriatric medicine.

Electronic equipment can transform the lives of some patients and their carers. Awareness by doctors, nurses, social workers and, sadly, even therapists of the modern range and potential of such equipment is often lacking. Both for the individual and caring teams, visits to Possum Controls Ltd. and the Disabled Living Foundation can increase understanding of the various ways that handicapped people can be helped.

REFERENCES

Department of Health and Social Security, 1983, "Arrangements for the
        Provision of Environmental Control and Communication Equipment through
        DHSS", HMSO, London.
Harris, A. I., Cox, E., and Smith, C., 1971, Handicapped and Impaired in
        Great Britain. Part 1., OPCS, HMSO, London.
Holden, T., 1980, Patiently Speaking, Nursing Times, June: 1035-1036.
Millard, P. H., and Smith, C. S., 1981, Personal Belongings,
        The Gerontologist, 21: 85-90.
Oliver, D. J., O'Gorman, B., and Saunders, C., 1986, Motor Neurone Disease,
        in: "Cash's Textbook of Neurology for Physiotherapists", P. Downie,
        ed., Faber and Faber, London.
Saunders, C., 1986, The Last Refuge, Nursing Times, Oct: 28-30.
St. Christopher's Hospice Information Service, 1986, Questionnaire: January,
        St Christopher's Hospice, London.
Wilkes, E., 1984, Dying Now, Lancet 1: 950-952.

SETTING UP A DISTRICT HEALTH AUTHORITY TERMINAL CARE SUPPORT TEAM

Richard Feinmann and Audrey Pointon

Stepping Hill Hospital
Stockport, U.K.

INTRODUCTION

Specialist teams in terminal care will hopefully become the norm in all District Health Authorities. Teams which are multi-disciplinary may provide better care, in that, a total district service can be encompassed and the service may be more acceptable to all health professionals. We describe the setting up of such a team and we believe that our experience will help others to proceed more quickly and efficiently.

DESCRIPTION

Over a period of about two years we have carefully planned a service for the terminally ill in Stockport. We have one of the largest hospices on the boundary on our district, but this provides a service for the whole of Greater Manchester. We also have six general and teaching hospitals within easy reach. However, no specialist service existed to help the terminally ill in their own homes. In Autumn 1984, we planned to provide such a service, linking the existing District General Hospital and Hospice care with the community. We were aware that there have been notable successes and failures (Bates et al. 1981; Herxheimer et al. 1985) in such services and we therefore, planned carefully to avoid these pitfalls.

Table 1.   INAUGURAL MEETING

Hospital Physician	Nurse Managers (4 D.H.A. Units)
Hospital Surgeon	District Nurse
Hospital Geriatrician	Senior Nurse Research and Development
Hospital Gynaecologist	
Three General Practitioners	Director of Social Services
Director of School of Nursing	Community Unit Administrator

Table 2.   TOPICS FOR CARE TEAM

---

(1) Definition and need in Health Authority

(2) Service required:
     Symptom control, support for relatives and patients, etc.

(3) Medical Input

(4) Nurse Input

(5) Social Worker Input and ? financing

(6) Nurse and Doctor education

(7) Nurse job description and financing

Table 3.   STOCKPORT TERMINAL CARE TEAM

Two full-time Macmillan Nurses

Hospital Consultant Physician

General Practitioner *

Retired Hospital Consultant*

Nurse Manager

---

* Also involved in local hospice

Our inaugural meeting was held in February 1985 and we invited professionals who would represent all fields of care in our district. (Table 1)

The idea of the service was enthusiastically received and Core Planning
Team Meetings were arranged over the following three months to report back
on various topics. (Table 2)

From these topics a draft document was produced, which was submitted
to the full meeting (Table 1) in May 1985. Once approved this document was
submitted to the District General Manager. Our team depended on funding for
two specialist Nurses, which we hoped would be funded for the first three
years by the National Society for Cancer Relief. The team (Table 3) consisted of professionals who could give support in the hospital, the hospice
and the community.

For the next year we became somewhat frustrated because health authorities do not move as quickly as enthusiasts might wish. Our document went
to and fro for consultation to the various interested groups. However, this
time was in fact, most valuable as it enabled us to sell our terminal care
service throughout the district. With the assistance, occasionally, of
drug companies, many of the Primary Health Care Teams were visited by us.
Often a short film on care of the dying was followed by a presentation of
our new service. Care was taken particularly with G.P.'s and District Nurses
to reassure them that the service was to help them, rather than interfere
and duplicate care. The various hospital division cogwheels were also
invited. A discussion in the Post-Graduate Department between Doctors

proved most useful and it became clear that although many professionals would use the service, many felt they already gave a good service. The seed was planted however, and we hoped that increasingly, Doctors and Nurses would use the service as it proved itself. Indeed, if there had been immediate acceptance by everyone, the Team could have been quickly inundated with requests.

By May 1986 the service had been accepted in principle by the Health Authority and the District General Manager wrote to the National Society for Cancer Relief requesting funding for our Macmillan Nurses. In July 1986 approval for the funding of the Nurses was obtained. No approval for the funding of a Social Worker and a Nurse Tutor for the School of Nursing was obtained although discussions with the N.S.C.R. and the Health Authority are still taking place.

To launch our services, a Multi-Disciplinary Symposium on Terminal Care was organised. This was chaired by the chairman of our District General Hospital. Experts gave their views of various topics and the Stockport Team Plan was presented in detail. By November 1986 the two Macmillan Nurses had been appointed and the service has been running for nine months. Much of the first three months, the two specialist Nurses spent introducing them-selves and re-selling the service to health professionals in the hospice, hospital and the community. The service is clearly still in its infancy, but we are pleased how well it has been accepted and used.

We hope that our experience will help persuade others to set up services of their own. We believe that a team which gives a service across the health authority is very worthwhile. Liaison and communication between the health professionals is improved and thus a service for patients can be developed so that care can be quickly arranged in which ever part of the health author-ity it is required. In particular, those patients who wish to be at home are not forgotten.

Careful planning of such a service is vital involving all health pro-fessionals. Education and communication which are an essential part of this planning must continue once the service is introduced.

REFERENCES

Bates, T., Clarke, D. G., Hoy, A. M. and Laird, P. P., 1981, The St Thomas' Hospital Terminal Care Support Team, Lancet.
Herxheimer, A., Begence , R., MacLean, R., Phillips, L., Southcott, B., and Walton, I., 1985, The short life of a Terminal Care Support Team: Experience of a Charing Cross Hospital, BMJ, 290.

A CREATIVE RESPONSE TO MULTIPLE LOSSES

David Frampton

St Joseph's Hospice
London, UK

Multiple losses characterise the closing stages of the lives of our patients who can no longer expect cure from medical intervention and have progressive disease. Losses such as the loss of job, loss of mobility, loss of status, loss of energy, dignity and control all tip the balance further against the patient, inducing an increased sadness and debility. Loss in itself can indeed cause physical pain as evidenced by a lady who wrote, "When I was five years old, my father died. He died of cancer. I have known for a long time he died of cancer, but not where the cancer was. Anyway wherever the cancer was the anguish it causes is the same. What devastation and destruction for the whole family. For me it was the end of the lucki-ness of having no memories of pain. Because truly, from then on, it was pain." At the age of 36, this lady was admitted to a hospice with severe pain which had proved very difficult to control. Reading her autobiography, however, revealed that she has had "pain" since the age of 5, pain clearly related to loss and augmented by the fact that she now has 3 children of junior school age, each with a different father, and so not only was she losing them but must have lost at least three men in the past. Clearly attention to her pain needed more than physical measures.

When talking about bereavement we are familiar with the many aspects of the process of loss which include anger, denial, bargaining, guilt, blame, questioning etc. Our patient who is suffering one loss after another as indicated above does not usually have time to come to terms with one loss before experiencing the next and as one patient said to me, "It's not so much a process of loss, but a battle ground." The impact of these losses can be such that the patient withdraws completely in an attempt to shut out the pain and as his or her personal sense of identity may well have been tied up with many of the things which have been lost, there may cease to be much obvious reason for staying alive. As one patient wrote -

Questions

What is the purpose of staying alive?
Why should I want to live?
What can I offer the world which surrounds me?
What can I hope to give?

I sat in the chapel and looked at the altar,
bleached white in the sunlights rays.

If God hears my questions he will answer
and rescue me from the maze -

Of self doubting, of sadness, of pain, and despair.

Please send understanding which I can share.

So the question we have to ask ourselves is, "What can we do with the pain which we cannot relieve?" Some people have attempted to produce diversional programmes for patients with cancer which are useful as far as they go but diversion does seem to suggest the idea of looking the other way while something nasty happens. Death is too important to be diverted from in this way all the time and a diversional programme may simply potentiate denial. It is also not appropriate to push patients into activity which they do not want; however, there is a fine dividing line between that and encouraging someone into an activity which they may well find gives them a new interest in living.

Dame Cicely Saunders has said, "You matter to the last moment of your life and we will do all we can not only to help you die peacefully but live until you die," but how much do we actually help our patients to live until they die? Indeed what is involved in living?

Maslow in 1945 talked about a hierarchy of needs which we all have. Shown in diagrammatic form as a pyramid this shows that the foundational needs have to be met first before the higher needs of love and esteem and self-actualisation can be met. (See Figure 1.)

Relating this to our dying patient we can adapt this diagram showing that having done all we can to support and help our patient there is still need for creative expression and fulfilment in some form or other. (See Figure 2.)

There are of course some patients who can, when their symptoms have been controlled and they are in a supportive environment, resume their previous interests and creative activities such as reading, letter writing, needle-work, painting etc. Some patients may need specific physical help to do some of these things such as the quadriplegic patient who may well need a page turning machine for his book. One paraplegic lady began to write poetry and

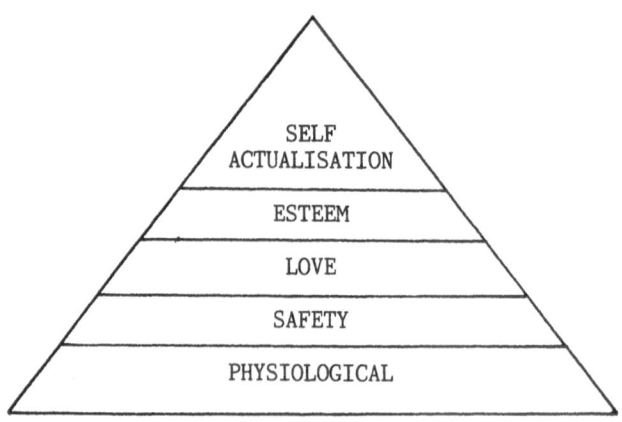

Figure 1.

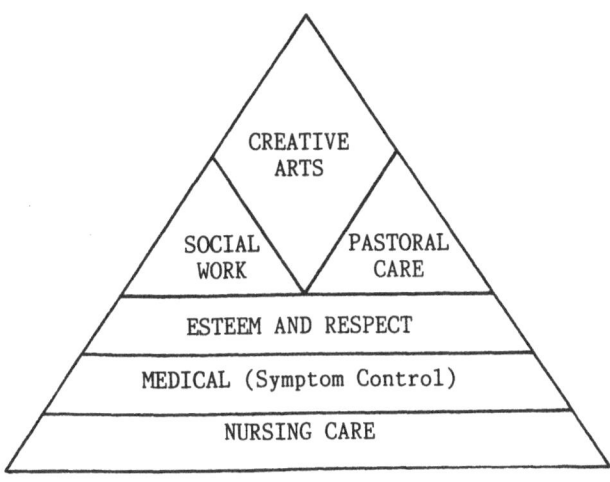

Figure 2.

she expressed in this poem her discovery that although she was grossly limited by her cancer in fact some other doors had been opened to her by her incapacity and she was able to walk through these in a very positive way.

1985

No thought of the body.
A healthy machine.
Needing:
Nourishment and sleep.
for a full, happy and busy life.

But clock watching, clock watching.

Suddenly, catastrophically,
cancer closes all previous doors.
Paralysed, half-aware,
emotionally and spiritually dead,
long days, long nights . . . .

Still clock watching, clock watching.

Slowly, through great skill and loving care,
the body becomes a manageable machine.
Through the selflessness of others,
there is a new freedom.

Freedom to develop family ties.
Renewing old friendships,
and the making of new.
Freedom from the petty tasks
of day to day living.

Time now for reading and writing.
Time now for laughing and crying.
Time now for praying.

The clock on the wall
is rarely consulted.

She has found new horizons as did another patient, already an accomplished
painter who in the closing two weeks of his life wanted to learn to paint
portraits. Help was provided in the shape of some magazine articles and to
his great joy he began his first portrait which though never completed gave
him the awareness of pushing on to new horizons despite, or even because of,
the limitations imposed by his illness.

Our patients can be helped to explore new horizons by taking them on
outings to local places of interest or by bringing in artistic performances
which they will probably not have had the opportunity of seeing before. The
project "Invitation to the Ballet" sponsored by Lederle Laboratories brought
a lot of new interest and excitement to patients when they visited the
hospice. Similarly regular visits from artists from the Council for Music
in Hospitals bring new experiences to patients. These concerts are often
held on the wards so that even weak patients who wish it can be involved in
the concerts while many of the items that are played will be familiar to at
least some of the patients. Often the instrument will not be well-known,
and seeing a harp played perhaps at the end of the bed or a beautifully
painted harpsichord accompanying a violin or flute brings a lot of joy and
some excitement too. Other performances such as flamenco dancers noticeably
increase the energy level in the ward.

Clearly one of the values of music is for reviving old memories and it
does seem to be important in the closing phases of life to remember back to
old experiences and somehow tie life together as a whole in order to be ready
to lay it down. In order to potentiate this we have introduced a violinist
and a flautist who play at the patients bedside, perhaps sitting on the bed
to play individually requested items which naturally stimulate conversation
about what these pieces mean to individual patients. Of course, permission
is sought from all patients within earshot of the music before this is em-
barked on, but often other relatives and patients are drawn into the conversation and musical reminiscence to the enjoyment and benefit of all.

Live music can of course not always be available and the portable
cassette players with light weight earphones are a real boon to the weak
patient and a library of many different types of taped music can be built up
so that the tastes of individual patients can be catered for.

Other things which stimulate reminiscence could well be encouraged such
as bringing pets into the hospice or making posies of herbs with patients.
Scent often has a powerful effect in stimulating reminiscence.

The question still remains as to whether it is possible to enable the
patients to be more active and creative themselves and indeed whether in
some way the pain of their many losses can itself be a creative stimulus.
It has been an aim of our arts programme to occupy time creatively not just
passively, in such a way to improve feelings of personal worth and purpose
at a time when life seems worthless and pointless.

One way of doing this can be to leave behind something of oneself, ones
own creation. In a way it reaches out for a sort of immortality but is also
a cherished legacy for the family. At a number of hospices, artists work
with patients to produce items of quality which can serve just such a
purpose. Fabric painting, basket weaving, jewellery making, painting and
other craft work can with skill on the artists part be very rewarding for a
patient who may never have tackled anything like it before. It is important
that the artist is aware of the patient's likely limitation of concentration
and weakness of limbs, but with careful provision and preparation of

materials superb results can be produced by inexperienced patients to everybody's great delight. If these creative tasks can be shared with a close
relative or friend 'bonding' is improved which is of considerable comfort
in bereavement.

At St Joseph's we have made particular use of poetry as we have a poet
in residence. Patients are encouraged as indicated in the previous poems to
commit their thoughts and feelings about their illness to paper, usually
this is not an activity they have tried before and a little encouragement
is needed but it is amazing how poignant are the poems which result. One
man was able to begin to say to his wife many of the things he had not felt
able to say over the years during the less than ideal marriage. His ability
to express his positive feelings for his wife in this way went a long way to
helping her through what was in any event a difficult bereavement time.

Our patients use the poetry to express their thoughts and feelings
about approaching death and many of the poems, particularly those about
adaptation to physical limitations and hospital life, can be very valuable
to give insight to the real needs of patients to their carers and to
students. On a lighter note this is demonstrated by the following poem.

Ode to a Commode

It isn't polite,
 and if
we could avoid it

How happy
 how happy we would be.

But now
 how shaming
How degrading.

What to do but try
 or try not to cry.

Perhaps
 we are too solemn.
Perhaps
 our dreary bodies
don't require
such emotion
devotion!

Please nurse .....
Please nurse .....
Please ....

Staff too of course are experiencing multiple losses and in consideration of their mental health and in the concern to do something about their
stress levels a creative response could also be considered. Art classes for
the staff or opportunities for staff to work with some of the artists
visiting patients etc, could well provide for this and at the same time help
them to realise the value which the arts can have for their patients.

The whole ambience of the hospice is important in this regard too. The
attractive and well thought out design and decoration of the environment
will stimulate creativity in both staff and patients. Nor should this
approach be limited to patients within the hospice or visiting the day
centre. Many patients in their own homes are trapped in the same dilemmas

and it is important that the components of home care should include hope inspiring strategies.

Naturally there is a variety of response to such opportunities for creative activity but it is surprising how much can be achieved and how much patients' spirits are raised by enthusiastic and sympathetic involvement with artists.

JUSQU'A LA MORT, ACCOMPAGNER LA VIE

Patricia Floriet

JAMALV
Grenoble, France

The French movement, "Jusqu'à la mort, Accompagner là vie" (Right up
to death, Accompanying life), lies directly in line with that of the Hospice
Movement. It has a particularity however in that many of the people
instrumental in creating the movement have never seen a hospice as such.
They have heard about them, read about them, even transmitted their teaching,
but it is almost impossible to open beds in France and our first palliative
care ward (Dr Abiven, Centre Hospitalier de la Cité Universitaire, Paris) is
only a few months old.

In France the idea of a 'mouroir', a place to die, is inacceptable to
most; as is often the idea of talking about death and, a priori, telling
someone he is about to die. Doctors hesitate to impart a diagnosis of
terminal illness. Nurses have not the right to 'tell'. If information is
given it is often to the spouse or to the children who carry it as a secret
cross, an impediment to natural communication. The dying patient is often
considered as a failure and embarrassing to the institution whose job is to
cure.

This seems an easy statement, a caricature maybe. It is not far from
the truth however and could probably be applied to many countries outside
the Anglo-Saxon world. It is, in any case, the situation with which many
members of JALMALV have been confronted and we feel that the history of our
experience could be of use to others who adhere to the philosophy of the
hospice movement but find it exceedingly difficult to put it into practice
in the context in which they live and work.

The JALMALV movement was founded in Grenoble, France, in June 1983,
the result of several months discussion among a dozen or so persons involved,
professionally or personally, with caring for the dying. René Schaerer,
oncologist, Janine Pillot, psychologist, and Christiane Jomain, nursing
training officer, were particularly conscious of the difficulties facing the
hospital carers, others were working professionally in different spheres:
Hospital,at home, community care for the elderly, private practice, social
work, counselling and teaching. Some of us had suffered personal bereavement,
most of us had had to cope with it in our work.

After several months discussion about our needs, our priorities and our
name we founded the movement, "Jusqu'a là Mort, Accompagner là Vie" in June
1983. These were our declared aims:

· To instigate and encourage research on the global needs of the dying.
· To contribute to the evolution of attitudes towards death.
· To give better and more comprehensive support to the dying, their families and their carers.
· To recognise for all of these, professionals and non-professionals, the need for training, counselling and time and space for discussion.
· To find with them the means.
· To contribute to the better care of the dying wherever they may be.
· To instigate and further the creation of a place wherein the dying can be openly welcomed and cared for and where, thanks to the close collaboration of nursing and medical staff, volunteers, clergy, families and friends, the aim would be to:

- take into consideration the total suffering of the patient according to its different elements: physical, moral,spiritual and social.
- take particular care to alleviate physical pain.
- find and teach better ways of treating and caring for the dying.

Globally we wanted to pinpoint the inadequacies of the care for the dying, make them more widely known to the people who could help.

Globally we wanted to tackle the problem on three levels:

to pinpoint the inadequacies of the existing structures;

to make them more widely known to those who could perhaps change things on a collective level - the deciders and the cash-givers;

to do what we could ourselves to provide answers to the individual needs of the frustrated or saddened carers.

A fourth area, that of creating a hospice as such, demanded much of our time in visits to the ministry of health, the regional and local representatives, hospital administrators et al. but led to little. We have for the moment put aside the idea in favour of more supple structures and the instillation of the hospice philosophy throughout institutional and community care through education and information, what we call in France: 'to sensitize'.

1983 was a time when there was a lot of talk of euthanasia and where possibilities of reanimation and medicated survival were becoming more and more prodigious - and costly. There was a lot of social movement around these two poles of thought and the argument was being presented as an alternative. On one side medicated survival and euthanasia, on the other death in pain, anguish and solitude. We were troubled, there must be some other way, some positive way of living one's death! We looked towards the work of the hospices. We read the literature (very little in French at that time), some of us travelled and gave talks on the hospices we had visited: Queen Victoria's in Montreal, Pilgrims' in Canterbury, St Joseph's and Trinity in London and general geriatric care in Britain.

We found better care for the dying but also more consideration for the carers, the recognition of need for training and counselling, time for discussion of feelings and reactions regarded as essential for coping with the difficult task of caring for the terminally ill.

We gradually worked out a strategy of monthly lectures on caring, coping, listening, touching, bereavement processes, spiritual needs, the integration of families into caring patterns, the potentialities of volunteers, etc., etc. We were present in public places, held a stand at the Forum of Associations and arranged a more widely publicised lecture by one of France's leading specialists in medical ethics, Patrick Verspieren, s.j. on "An Alternative to Euthanasia?".

At the request of our members we organised short and on-going courses on listening and counselling, touching and massage, the understanding of bereavement, medication and the specific demands of terminal care. Members of the organisation are often asked to give talks to hospital and community carers in the towns around and to students in training colleges and schools.

We brought out a quarterly publication to take up these themes. Our subscribers, at first from Grenoble and Chambéry, its neighbour, started coming from all over France. We put subscribers in touch with each other so that they could get together. Several groups asked for lecturers, attracted wider attention and set up local JALMALV groups in their turn.

We have now established a National Federation of JALMALV and Associated Groups. It is based on the associations in Besançon, Chambéry, Dijon, Grenoble, Montpellier, Nice and Vierzon but already joined by Auvergne, Touraine and Pays de la Loire and other groups desirous to adhere to our declaration of intent which now includes a further passage to better define the meaning we give to the word "accompaniment":

"For the federation, the accompaniment of the dying and the palliative care involved must give the dying person and his entourage the possibility of living through the end of his life, neither hastening the end nor pro-longing life by unremitting medication."

We feel it essential that the Federation does not enclose groups into the name of JALMALV but leaves space for many other organisations often previous to our own who are doing similar work following the same aims in order to create a movement of national impetus capable of inducing change.

Membership is currently around 2000 people coming from all walks of life, feeling personal and professional concern about terminal care: cancer sufferers, the elderly, their families, voluntary and professional carers, hospital and health administrators, teachers, clergy, students etc.

We are having great difficulty answering the demand for training, speaking, writing, while each pursuing our professional roles, already very demanding. We are more and more working with the established educational actors in order to sensitize the trainers wherever they be. We intervene in university and adult education courses for medical and nursing carers, gerontologists, health administrators, hoping that our message will have an influence on organisation and be of benefit to more people. We have even answered demands from Belgium and Luxembourg and we are represented here, in US and Canada to learn and to manifest our need of solidarity.

We are hoping that there will soon be a possibility of joining up with those working in this direction in the rest of Europe and we are ready to co-ordinate initial processes of getting to know each other by publishing addresses and actions in our bulletin. Our means are small but the world is large. New caring criteria must be suggested and the means must be found, otherwise the dying will continue to be at the wrong end of social priorities.

There is no hospice movement in France and just one 'hospice' - but the impulse has been given, the people are becoming more conscious of need and a government writ as been circulated to all hospitals to ask the admini- strators to set up steering committees to examine the local situation and more recently the care of the dying has been introduced into the syllabus of medical studies. Community care teams for the elderly are being asked to care for younger adults wishing to die in their home. The work is under way and, in part, thanks to the different associations in Paris and in the provinces who spare no effort in their work.

SELF HELP AND THE ROLE OF PSYCHOSOCIAL SUPPORT AND THERAPY

Milly Jolley

PLUS Self-Help Association
Edinburgh, U.K.

On diagnosis, the cancer patient is presented immediately with a number of problems – the stigma, the following isolation, the possibility of terminal illness with cancer at some time, the possibility of severe pain, the need for treatment which may be traumatic, mutilating, nauseating or disabling in its side effects. With these may follow family disruption, financial repercussions with life style changes. Though all these may not impinge at once, the cancer patient knows on diagnosis that life will never be the same again.

The negative connotations of the word 'cancer' seem to be resistant both to the evidence of the availability of more effective treatment for some forms, and to the more open policy of communication in existence today. The feelings relate to patients, family, friends and Health Care Professionals alike. Cancer remains a threat to the medical profession in respect to control of the disease (Rosser and Maguire, 1982). The emotional reaction to cancer and its recurrence provides the same cultural framework for all. The category into which the cancer falls (i.e. good, fair, poor prognosis) undoubtedly influences the outcome at the onset; not only in respect of the disease in the patient and the response to it but also by the reaction of the carers, professionals and family (Greer, Morris and Pettingale, 1979).

Self help does help. It was to break this circle of negativity that the self help group PLUS was formed by four cancer patients seven years ago – to create by means of mutual support an environment of a positive nature wherein the self could add something of its own – and if invited could become a member of the interdisciplinary team.

The multidisciplinary team is essential to the patient to assess the value of, and the need for continuation of treatment, the necessity for ancillary programmes of care, the nursing arrangements, the stability of the home situation, the emotional balance and the spiritual direction. But the patient needs a personal life however brief the span is to be, and help to achieve it. The recognition of the team of the value of self help, and of the self help group, would add psychosocial support of a new kind to cancer therapy.

Needs of cancer patient focus primarily on reassurance of worth, the right of personal responsibility for dignity, and an opportunity for self discovery – according to our experience within the group – especially when moving towards death. New perceptions can come very quickly leading to growth of the person; enabling this to be said "I would not go back to being what I was. I would not have things any other way". Handled in a proper way for the patient, there is a 'rightness' about death, comforting to the patient, consoling to the family and enriching to friends. In PLUS experience - socialisation in its broadest sense of making loving relationships, giving and receiving affection, can be done to the last days.

The wellbeing of the cancer patient depends on being understood. The needs are well defined - good communication, information as required, personal involvement with decisions, honest relationships with professionals, time, privacy, and continuity of care, access to other resources and kin support. Many of these cause problems and are interrelated depending specifically on two - time and tendency towards distancing (Maguire, 1975).

Distancing may be a time saving technique, or a protective barrier. The patient for whom nothing more can be done is easily passed by on a ward, or dismissed with an ambiguous phrase at appointment. This is perfectly, painfully recognisable to the patient. The private word is a word valued, and relates to the need for a personal relationship which may not always be the medical member of the team. From the patient's point of view interviews are rushed, difficult questions cannot be articulated, information asked for not always given, the questions brushed aside. Alternatively the quite direct answer comes over as brutal or unnecessarily frank and the patient not recovered from the shock before out of the door. These sorts of interviews, especially when the patient is told terminal unexpectedly, are brooded over and recounted with distress sometimes many years later. The patient seeks for a reason, a cause of the disease (Pinell, 1982). One quote from a member, "I think professionals' attitudes must change so that they treat us as equals - during crises we are vulnerable. We are desperate for help. But we are not fools, and if we co-operate through better understanding of what it's all about surely this is better for everyone." Patients generally complain about lack of support after bad news, particularly those without family present. Information requested most frequently concerns drug reactions, the need for, and results of, investigations.

Our members speak of a need to know more and to be reassured, to be allowed hope. Even with the terminal patient these are not incompatible. It should always be possible to reassure about forthcoming support, about relief of pain, to demonstrate recognition of the traumatic situation, with loving kindness, however pressed.

Continuity of care is difficult to achieve for the staff but a requirement of the patient. The isolation and subsequent loss of self esteem relate to the stigma, and to the succession of professionals involved of necessity in cancer treatment. An ongoing relationship as 'friend', professional or otherwise is vital. To combat isolation there must be at least one person who knows the facts, understands the occasions of panic and despair, is not judgemental, who will support during treatment and afterwards - available between appointments and checkups - who will not turn away from unrelieved pain and is able to watch death approach with equanimity. The underlying security reduces anxiety, and depression, and counteracts isolation by removing stigma. It will not necessarily present projection of anger, or denial but does enable movement to be made towards acceptance. With full acceptance, it sometimes happens that patients live much longer than expected; useful lives which have quality and meaning, for themselves and others.

The question is - is it possible for professionals to allow, sustain and continue to make, such close personal relationships with a succession of dying patients? PLUS has explored the possibility of providing the required support and continuity of care on a non-professional basis, using the experiences of membership in different ways of coping with disease (Clement-Jones, 1985), at the same time giving patients involvement with the management of their own illness. It seeks to provide a suitably positive environment for developing a new lifestyle which enables the person to continue to the end - providing means for activity often denied by an over protective family and tailored to the individual out of knowledge of support needs and last wishes of the dying patient.

An outline of PLUS will give a background to show how a self help group can work effectively. My paper 'Community Care and Self Help' is available with detail. PLUS Edinburgh, is an organisation for people with cancer and others in pain - a mixed group lessens the stigma immediately. In PLUS the member is also the volunteer and vice versa. All members can contribute something and it is accepted that all volunteers have problems of some sort (usually it is bereavement). PLUS was a house group in 1980 which grew rapidly, became a charity in 1984 and now has offices, a drop-in centre and evening venues and six paid part-time staff, two groups in West Lothian, and contacts all over Scotland.

Transport to a variety of activities and opportunities for social contacts, both afternoon and evening, make it possible for the frail and housebound to join in. Sick members are matched to car and driver. Valuable friendships ensue. Active participation in events is encouraged and leads to rapid rehabilitation in an unthreatening atmosphere (Hammer, 1983). The terminally ill find it possible to interact; help remain independent, and give support to others. In PLUS there is no passive recipient. The bereaved find it easy to get the support they need to continue normal roles (Thomson, 1979). The networking, which is extensive, is especially valuable to those with no relatives and few friends. For two the centre is considered as a second home! Three require our advocacy. The telephone is used as a communication tool. It serves the network and is used by the severely ill and very handicapped, most often during evenings and weekends. It is most valued by those alone and by carers. It offers choice and control for those who have little opportunity to exercise either. Paradoxically for the 'unsatiables' its availability reduces the constant desperate need to call for help.

This mutual sharing meets the needs of the whole person - practical, emotional and spiritual. The relationships are much closer than professional ones. The network is held together by common experience and common purpose (Robinson, 1978). The sense of unity is often felt collectively by a shared silence which falls spontaneously with expression of grief or loss, a peak group experience. The terminally ill are supported by this kind of happening. The dying like to know they will be missed. Within the group they know it will be so. The loss of members by death does not prove to be a harrowing experience. The richness of the relationship, being instead, reward.

Our terminally ill, who knit or raise funds in other ways, organise an appeal, share in intercessionary prayer, support others in like or unlike situations from bed or wheelchair, by phone or letter, continue to use their knowledge and experience. These are loved and loving, valuable and valued, productive and growing beyond every conventional expectation. Their courage becomes a resource to the community in itself.

PLUS principles have been carefully worked out. Members have pain from organic illness, or care for someone, or their bereavement relates to it. The aim is the growth of the person which PLUS sees as coming about by change (Lock, 1986). The base is friendship, which accepts people as they are, so that they may be themselves without pretence. The maintenance of loving relationships between all individuals, whether members or staff is its essence. Friendship is given and received in a measure relative to the capacity of the person and their desire for it. Contributions of help and in kind are accepted and received as relative to the capacity of the individual to give, and their responsibilities; and as being of equal value. Practical help in difficulties is given and taken on a constructive basis. PLUS does not advise unless there are exceptional circumstances; but supplies information on request which is carefully checked and regularly updated. Confidentiality is respected. Only details necessary for mailing are recorded. Case records are not kept. These principles have been expanded into guidelines for members and volunteers.

Hospice and hospitals are visited by PLUS friends. Not many members look towards the hospice. Once there, members are available to the hospice team. Hospitals welcome PLUS visits especially to the terminally ill with no relatives. PLUS supplements home help services on occasions, covers weekend emergencies at times of bed shortages or when the patient prefers to remain at home. In this way PLUS can provide the continuity of care required by the patient, support for a carer (especially for one in difficulties) and later for the bereaved. It also provides advocacy where required and requested.

Statistics are based on figures for May 1987. PLUS membership has been pruned twice in the past year, leaving 203 families. Pruned means removal of those who have left or died. Some leave because they have recovered, others because they do not find what they want for a variety of reasons. Often these remain on the periphery, glad we are there, and make an occasional phone call and continue to help others. A few leave and return as health fluctuates. Membership includes sick, carers, bereaved and well helpers with appropriate motivation. The latter are mainly drivers – drivers providing 25% of the total. PLUS provided 1502 car journeys last year mainly to centre and evening activities, social outings, with occasional supported shopping, or emergency hospital arrangements. Of the 114 really sick and disabled using our transport system, 50% are cancer related and 20% of these have a second major health problem. All our six terminal members are cancers. Few families with cars use them for transport of their disabled to PLUS activities, due to the need for respite, nevertheless our system is not exploited. The system is free but voluntary donations are often made: independence being a matter of pride, it is sometimes necessary to persuade our impaired and restricted mobility group to accept assistance. Membership is 80% female, women being less supported than men. 16% of total membership requires support through bereavement, half of these being cancer deaths. Members frequently fit into more than one category e.g. a cancer patient with a major secondary illness is a carer. The spouse is dependent.

Counselling for the terminal cancer patient is a major requirement. This is done by means of a weekly discussion group where death (aspects of dying) is an acceptable topic, and on a one to one basis, with home visits if requested. The carer is the second most needy group. The carer normally seeks a private word, anxious to do the right thing. The telephone is often the most convenient way of contact. In bereavement the carer usually comes back for immediate support, but does not return (or join) as a helper until some grief is worked through.

Staff and volunteer relationships present some problems. In areas of management, difficulties arise where volunteers are called upon to do the complex organisational work required; and when there is need for a paid post before funding is available for it. In fact the funding of voluntary bodies working in conjunction with statutory bodies is an important issue leading to the collapse of some self help groups when key figures are not available on a voluntary basis. The use of paid staff to ensure continuity is essential. The heart of the self help group is its experience of illness, especially of cancer, and the illness does take its toll: The supporting volunteers bring all the problems of volunteering with the additional one of ongoing illness. A number of fit volunteers with the right motivation is essential. Where staff have background experience of relevant concerns, the difficulties are minimised. Their willingness to do some voluntary work in addition, gives insights to them and the members which are useful.

Training also presents some difficulty due to the varied nature of the membership. Drivers often being bereaved, have experience of transport arrangements for the frail terminally ill. They are all offered simple training in first aid and lifting techniques, and monthly meetings to share experience. Outside training for counselling has been used but not filled the needs. We shall provide our own training scheme based on our self help experience with cancer, to start in the Autumn. It will be offered to staff and volunteers. Staff and volunteers are encouraged to make use of general training programmes available, and a grant was obtained for this purpose. Such training will make the acceptance of members of selp help groups easier for multidisciplinary teams. In fact members often already have health care professional qualifications and enjoy using their skills in a different ambiance.

The expectation and achievement in self help groups varies. The expectation varies relating to the capacity of the individuals and the severity of incapacity in illness. At its lowest it fills the role of a club where social intercourse can be taken or left at will, without obligation. This is useful and non threatening, suits passive and aggressive individuals alike, is acceptable to the very ill and also those using it to 'try out' before returning to normal activity. This mix is useful in itself.

At its best personality 'flowers' and there is spiritual growth. The expectation here is for appreciation of the struggle and the recognition of the growth, and for loving interchange.

There is also the expectation of helpful guidance, a sharing of techniques, particularly in regard to pain; and of support by understanding and by practical means. It is important that there is always someone there, at the end of a telephone line - and that it is not demeaning to avail oneself of it and that someone is capable of responding (Lock, 1986). Lastly and most difficult, is the expectation of being given strength in the later phases of illness. When expectation is accompanied by growth it can always be filled. The members own strength sharing the burden. The more growth, the more support available. At a certain point the giving becomes mutual. The dying have something to give. The achievement varies as much as the expectation but it is not related to the illness but to the capacity of the individual to change. One of the many factors which cumulatively cause illness is an inability to change with changed circumstances. PLUS offers a new chance, new friends, somewhere new to change in. The amount of change is dependent upon the amount of improvement which can be tolerated in relation to other factors of the illness.

In conclusion, the self help group, using PLUS experience, is shown to be a valuable psychosocial support in therapy and outwith it, for the terminal cancer patient. It is an asset to the multidisciplinary team in its support, and in enabling the patient to contribute to it. The role of the group in providing continuity of care for the whole person is demonstrated, as is its part in community care. A case is made for the recognition of the value of self help groups in assisting patients 'to remain persons' in their own eyes, with lives of quality and significance, even to the last days.

REFERENCES

Clement-Jones, V., 1985, Cancer and beyond: the formation of BACUP, <u>B.M.J.</u>, 291:1021.

Greer, S., Morris, T. and Pettingale, K. W., 1979, Psychological response to breast cancer: effect on outcome, <u>Lancet</u>, 2(8146):785-7.

Hammer, M., 1983, 'Core' and 'extended' social networks in relation to health and illness, <u>Soc. Soi. Med.</u>, 17:405-411.

Lock, S., 1986, Self help groups: the fourth estate in medicine?, <u>B.M.J.</u>. 293:1596-1599.

Maguire, P. 1985, Barriers to psychological care of the dying, <u>B.M.J.</u>, 291:1711-1713.

Pinell, P., 1982, How do cancer patients express their points of view? <u>Sociology of Health and Illness</u>, 9:25-44.

Robinson, D., 1979, Self help groups, <u>Br.J.Hosp.Med.</u>, 20(3):306-11.

Rosser, J. E. and Maquire, P., 1982, Dilemmas in general practice; the care of the cancer patient, <u>Soc.Soi.Med.</u>, 16:315-332.

Thomson, I., 1979, "Dilemmas of Dying", Edinburgh University Press, U.K.

SHORT-TERM PSYCHOTHERAPY AND CRISIS INTERVENTION IN BEREAVEMENT

Francesco Campione and Nadia Crotti

Dipartimento di Psicologia
Bologna, Italy

In Italy, probably due to the particular organization of medical assistance, the tendency is to clearly distinguish between interventions characteristic of the initial phase of bereavement marked by acute emotional suffering, and those peculiar to subsequent phases, characterized by chronic emotive sufferance some times even in the form of psychopathologic symptoms. This differentiation roughly corresponds to two different ways of conceiving loss typical of every bereavement. The loss may, in fact, be considered: a) as a stressing event whose emotional seriousness may be evaluated in the same way of any other stressing event by means of quantitative scale; b) as an event the sense of which derives from the biographic events of the libido, the now lost object of love being one of the goals of the subject's libidinal investment.

The differentiation as to the manner of conceiving the loss coincides with the difference in organizing and accomplishing the psychological assistance intervention for bereaved people.

So, by following the first approach, one tends to help the subject spontaneously seeking an efficient coping pattern that will make him overcome the distress. Such an intervention is very similar to that called "crisis intervention" and is realized in Italy mainly through psychotropic drugs prescribed by the general practitioner or, less frequently, by the psychiatrist. If, instead, the second approach is preferred, an attempt will be made to help the subject elaborate the bereavement, that is, withdraw from the lost loved one by removing the obstacles usually represented by defensive mechanisms tending unsuccessfully to cancel forbidden impulses, feelings of guilt, unbearable distress, basic conflicts, etc. from one's conscience.

This type of intervention utilizes the applications of short-term psychotherapy according to the experience patterns acquired and has only recently been put into practice in Italy due to historical reasons (among them the persisting diffidence of the predominant psychoanalytic school to short-term psychotherapies, the forces that tend to preserve the collective rituals of approach in regional cultures to the situation of bereavement).

In planning a psychotherapeutic intervention procedure to assist bereaved persons, we were struck by the precise coincidence in literature (Bowlby, 1982; Parkes, 1972; Parkes and Weiss, 1983; Volkan, 1981; Raphael, 1984), between the two conceptions present in our context and the two therapeutic procedures, crisis intervention and short-term psychotherapy.

Starting from this, we gradually acquired awareness of the need to adequately work this field, to clarify the concept of crisis. Broad and restricted definitions have been found in the literature (Sifneos, 1979); Caplan, 1974), but non specifically referring to the particular situations of bereavement. We then returned to observation of reality continuing to use the two parameters (cognitive, and psychoanalytical) present in our cultural context and mentioned above.

If we assume that the two conceptions exclude each other, we can say: I) Bereavement crisis may be understood as an acute stress for the subject, for his decisional capacity, his self-esteem and his adjustment until an efficient coping strategy lowers his emotive tension; II) the loss will bring about a crisis of the subject's libidinal economy resulting in chronic emotive suffering. In the first case, the bereaved needs help because an acute stress prevents him from living, while, in the second, the bereaved party needs help due to the loss of the loved one, thus preventing him from continuing to love.

Actually the two conceptions do not cancel each other since cases exist where the reaction to loss seems to be mainly an acute crisis or a chronic one; but situations are met with where both are present together and are reciprocally cleared up (we shall return to this with the analysis of two clinical cases). To our way of thinking, this leads to the need to overcome, as being partial, the two bereavement crisis conceptions just illustrated.

One could say that there is a need to set up a psychosomatic conception of bereavement, where the psychoneurologic and psychodynamic aspects can find greater integration. To this end, we have begun to check the hypothesis of conceiving bereavement crisis as existential, a crisis as De Martino (1975) would say of presence. In other words, a serious loss would be conceived as a crisis of the meaning of existence, which may be expressed mainly in psychoneurologic or psychodynamic terms, depending on the subject's identity, a crisis which, however, always expresses the affected existence (Campione, 1986).

In this sense, stress, behaviour and symptoms (normal or pathological) would be considered 'expressions' of different level and style of the exist-ential crisis caused by loss. On these lines we have prepared a model of intervention to assist the bereaved persons by helping them to regain the meaning of life upset by the loss, with the double acceptation of restoring the lost meaning and the search for a new one. In this model, crisis inter-vention and short-term psychotherapy, become integrated, since in any case, the aim of the assistance is in terms of existential meanings of all express-ions of his crisis. Where acute emotional stress dominates, it is clearly impossible to bring the subject to understand its meaning without helping him to ease the tension, though, as we know, explaining is one of the most important factors towards efficient coping with respect to an emotionally negative situation.

On the other hand, neurotic crystallization of the crisis (a phobia, for instance), based on a shifting of meaning in order to reduce emotive suffering, cannot be overcome without bringing the subject back to the grief he did not want to suffer (think to the cases where, in order to let the griefwork begin, the mourning subject must accept the pain of the loss suffered).

An integral part of this model is the extensive use made of the concept of bereavement. We have, in other words, conceived as bereavement not only the existential expressions of the loss of a relative, but also those of: the loss of a part (physical or psychic) of oneself or of a dear one.

Finally, a feature of this model, besides the short duration of psycho-therapeutic intervention, is the consideration of all expressions of the existential crisis of bereavement as equally significant and equally partial. From this, every expression is placed in context with respect to a wider background to be reconstructed empathically: the sense on which the manner of being of everyone is based!

We are therefore dealing with an intervention on bereavement situation which acknowledges the validity of all approaches (considering each as corresponding to some particular expression of the existential crisis due to bereavement) and, at the same time, attempts to integrate them in seeking an overall cultural solution specific for every existential crisis.

The psychologist is the central figure in this model, his task being to co-ordinate the team, bringing the intervention of all the other members (the psychiatrist, the social worker, the general practitioner, the priest, etc.) back to the sense context of the interested existence. The psychological approach can, in this, attempt to compensate certain weakened social function by triggering a socio-cultural process modifying the environmental context in which the personal crisis of the bereaved person occurs.

We shall now briefly analyse two clinical cases to concretely illustrate our model and its possibilities.

1. A.M., age 43, female: removal and immediate reconstruction of the breast. The operation causes the patient acute distress and she goes to the psychiatrist who was already treating her, to ask for supplementary drugs. The psychiatrist points out the limits of the pharmacological approach and sends the patient to the psychologist to whom the patient makes the same kind of request.

   The case is typical: most people requesting help for an acute emotional crisis, also bring a suggestion on the tendential coping modality. In this case, the patient knows only the well-tried pharmacological coping and would like to intensify the efficacy in the presence of an acute emotive crisis. In the frame of our intervention procedure, after careful assessment of the case, aimed to evaluating the gravity of the emotional stress so as to be in a position to give an adequate response to the patient's request, we try to empathically understand its expressive meaning. In other words, we ask: in what manner is this person, through his emotive suffering and his coping patterns, expressing his way of being in the world, the existential meaning on which she based his existence? For this purpose the psychologist suggests: we meet a certain number of times in concomitance with medical checks in the institute (in this case the work is done in an institute for the treatment of tumors). With the first meeting the case begins to clear up. The patient says: "I'm sorry, I'm so silly. I'm ill and have nothing to tell you". But when the psychologist invites her to talk about her current life situation there emerges a feeling of inadequacy: "I can no longer breast feed or be fed", she says. And she tells the story of her relationship with a brother who died at 13, with whom she played at feeding and being fed. She then adds it is her husband who nourishes her now, warm, calm and protective.

   To be brief, we would say that our approach permitted the patient's call for help to be interpreted correctly, not as an acute crisis due mainly to the contingency of the loss and reconstruction of the breast, but as acute renewal of a chronic crisis due to a previous bereavement not overcome: the loss of the brother that had placed her identity in crisis as sister capable of 'breast feeding' him and of being fed by him. The breast cancer emphasizes this situation causing an acute existential crisis, the re-edition of the chronic one. The immediate reconstruction of the breast suggests to the patient a denial of the loss suffered ("You have a new breast, just as if you had never lost it!"). This underlines the patient's regressive ways of reacting to the situation, so neither the drugs she takes nor the husband who 'feeds' her are enough any more.

The psychological intervention suggests another way to her, through which the patient expresses her constant problem, understands that the old breast and the new are equivalent, can 'confess' to her husband the 'incestuous' love for her brother and when, after this, it is the husband who falls into crisis (he can't sleep any more) the patient begins to see a new possibility in the meaning of existence, a more adult way of loving her husband and being loved by him, which permit her in the end to return to work, that is, to reinvest the world again.

We have mentioned this case to show how in our model an acute crisis can be explained and overcome by inserting it in a sense context of which at the same time it is one of the expressions.

Equally interesting is the second case exemplifying those situations where it is necessary to 'go back' to an acute crisis not before experienced in order to understand and overcome a neurotic reaction to a serious loss;

2. A.B., 35 years old, female, lost a son of 11 due to a grave form of leukemia.

She comes after two years of trying to get over her grief at the loss of her son by following a strategy suggested by the family environment and characterized by the invitation to forget and distract herself by working, travelling, and so on. She suffers from symptoms of nocturnal anxiety (sudden wakening with tachycardia and dysnoea). The patient appears to share the coping strategy spontaneously effected by the family and tends to distort and minimize the episodes of nocturnal anxiety (she takes some psychotropic drug).

She would like to succeed in carrying out the strategy that her husband and her daughter manage perfectly, but she cannot: she always thinks of her son, is depressed, etc. That is why she comes, to be helped in this only strategy she consciously considered possible.

Deeper investigation of the case brings together the re-awakening and nocturnal anxiety through precise nightmares (she always dreamt of her son in the worst period, when his body was deformed and suffering). The evaluation is that we are in presence of a traumatic neurosis in a Freudian sense (Freud, 1977), that is, in the presence of a coercive pathological defence against the acceptance of her son's death by a continuous return to the phase preceding death. The neurotic symptom expresses the patient's impossibility to accept her son's death, which she tries to do remaining fixed at the terminal phase, but she is incapable of succeeding because she would then relive her son's death every night, waking up a moment before he died or at the moment in which she is about to relive the death she refuses. However, the neurotic symptom also has the secondary advantage of allowing her to continue suffering for her son, which its environmental context with its tendency to forget, would not permit. Besides, the neurotic symptom allows the patient to express the ambivalence towards this son that she had not wanted, though she came to accept him, through a reparatory attitude, that is, by taking great care of him during infancy and even more so during his illness. The patient cannot speak of all this to anyone, just as she is unable to follow her spontaneous tendency to see the films of her son's life, because she consciously shares the family coping strategy.

The purpose of psychotherapy in this case was formulated in a precise focus: the son's death, places this woman's sense of existence in crisis expressed thus in the patient's own words: "When someone I know is in a state of need I must do something for him. This sometimes exhausts me but I can't help it"; so it was necessary to help this woman to accept her son's death which could specifically mean: a) find a way to continue to have a reparatory attitude towards him, that is to try to 'repare' his death, too; b) reconstruct the sense of her manner of being with a new strategy of managing her guilt sentiments. The two ways are both present in patient's world and really constitute the poles of her conflict. The first is the way to identify herself with her son to interiorize him as an object protected and pacified to the point of no longer feeling the sense of guilt towards him: the second way opens when the patient says of herself: "Sometimes I fear I am completely wrong and ought to think of myself and nothing else".

Psychotherapy in this case allowed removal in three months the obstacle of ambiental coping strategy which made the patient repress her sorrow for her son's death, suggesting it was unbearable. In this way the patient was able to accede to her grief at the loss of her son; she wept for him a long time, was upset by a long emotive crisis, after which the bereavement process began, and little by little, the patient was able to recover everything positive about her son, the meaning of the son who died for her. She was able to identify herself with him, interiorize him and make his loss a reason for strengthening her way of being oblational and protective towards her husband and daughter.

The decisive moment came when the patient said "I thought the death of my son should have a meaning and I couldn't find it, rather did it call into question the meaning of everything, the existence and goodness of God too. Then I understood that even though it remains absurd how a child can die, for me the death of my son may have a much deeper meaning. I understand now that a mother who has lost a child is a better mother for the child that remains, because she loves him in a more mature way, now that she knows that a son may be loved even if he no longer lives, even though one can expect nothing more from him".

REFERENCES

Bowlby, J., 1982, Attachment and loss: retrospect and prospect, American Journal of Ortopsychiatry, 52:664-678.
Campione, F., 1986,'Guida all'Assistenza Psicologica del Malato Grave' (Ama il prossimo tuo come se stesso), Patron, Bologna.
Caplan, G.,1964,'Principles of Preventive Psychiatry',Basic Books,New York.
De Martino, E., 1975, 'Morte e Pianto Rituale',Boringhieri, Torino.
Freud, S., 1977, Aldila del principio del piacere, in 'Opere', Boringhieri, Torino.
Parkes, C. M., 1972, 'Bereavement Study of Grief in Adult Life', International University Press, New York.
Parkes, C. M., and Weiss, R. W., 1983, 'Recovery from Bereavement', Basic Books, New York.
Raphael, B., 1984, 'The Anatomy of Bereavement', Hutchinson, London.
Sifneos, P. E., 1979, 'Short-term Dynamic Psychotherapy', Plenum, New York.
Volkan, V., 1981, 'Linking Object and Linking Phenomena: A Study of the forms, symptoms, metapsychology and therapy of complicated mourning, International Universities Press, New York.

ACKNOWLEDGEMENT

The research was supported by CNR (Oncology) Contract n.8600338V4

A FAMILY AND A TEAM - NURSES' ROLES IN IN-PATIENT TERMINAL CARE

Nicky James

Institute of Health Care Studies
University College of Swansea
Swansea, U.K.

The adaptions of principles when they are put into practice is both
hopeful and challenging. Hopeful because it means that those involved are
actively participating in making principles relevant to their own circumstances. Challenging because of the need to ensure that the adaptions
enhance the principles on which they were based, building on them rather
than detracting from them.

The links between 'family' and 'team' which provide the title of this
essay come from the way the terms were used by nurses during a participating
observation study of a Continuing Care Unit in the north-east of Britain.
One of the results of this ethnographic study was that in combination, the
'family' and 'team' help explain how the nurses perceived their roles. The
tensions between 'family' and 'team' which are exposed through the nurses use
of them, contribute to an understanding of the potential and effectiveness of
these principles in public service.

PRINCIPLES

The critique of terminal care which developed during the 1960's and
1970's revealed problems with the quality and delivery of the care of the
dying. Once untreated pain and discomfort and the impersonality of terminal
care were identified as factors affecting the quality of life before death,
plans to alleviate them could be developed. The provision of family care
through interdisciplinary teamwork has become a significant organisational
strategy in attempting to remedy the institutional impersonality of terminal
care.

Family

Notions of 'family' are integral to the principles of good terminal
care and although the definition of 'family' is not specified it tends to be
used in an idealised form. The specification that 'the family is the unit
of care' has been internationally adopted by hospices (Saunders, 1976; Parkes,
1978; Lack, 1983) and takes account of the ill-person as a social being with
a life and significance beyond the confines of their illness.

In addition those involved in the care of the dying, paid staff,
volunteers and friends have been encouraged to judge standards of care by

reference to their own family – what would my brother/mother/father/grand-mother like in these circumstances, and how would I react if that were me? Thus reference to the carers own family sets the standard of good terminal care, with the vital addition of the highest quality professional knowledge and skills.

Early on Saunders wrote of offering to 'be the family' of an ill-person who was otherwise alone, and thereby committed herself to an involvement with the patients. Formerly involved caring had been considered bad practice within an 'objective', 'rational' system of health care, the overt explana-tion being that it would interfere with clear and effective treatment.

Thus 'family' has been used in 3 ways in hospice care:

- family as the unit of care
- reference to the carers own family as a means of assessing the standards of care
- acting in addition to or a stand-in for the patients own family, and thereby developing close, warm relationships of trust and friendship.

In each of these expressions of 'family care', sentiment and emotion are given a centrality in the process of life before and after death both for the carer and those cared for.

Team

In the United States the National Hospice Organisation identified the core members of the team as being the patient/family unit, the primary physician, the nurse, social worker, volunteers, and the clergy (Hadlock, 1983), and thus echoed Lamerton's earlier prescription for 'teamwork' in Britain (Lamerton, 1973). Within this definition of the team, the family becomes one part of a larger whole working towards the single goal, 'euthanatos' (Twycross, 1973). Narrower definitions of the team refer to professional multi-disciplinary or inter-disciplinary teams, whose task is to use their joint expertise in the management of 'total pain'. Other more limited 'teams' have developed when a service is based on a single disci-pline, for instance a nursing facility which calls in auxiliary help from doctors, social workers, clergy and other professionals when it is thought necessary.

Though the composition of 'teams' has varied enormously in different parts of the world and within each country, in principle their structure and function has been that of a group involved in a single purpose. Members meet regularly to review progress and thereby share their different per-spectives and skills. In principle a consequence of the development of what Lamerton refers to as 'a partnership of equals' (Lamerton, 1973) is the 'role blurring' mentioned by Hadlock (1983), with the contributions of each discipline valued, and enough information made available to all disciplines to avoid the fragmentation of care which formerly led to poor communication and poor patient care.

The hope of 'teamwork' lay in its singleness of purpose and in learning to give individual care tailored to the needs of each ill-person and their family. The challenge offered by such an idea of 'teamwork' was how to develop and maintain it, for the majority of the paid staff had been trained in organisations geared to coping systematically with large numbers of people, and riven with inter and intra-disciplinary divisions. For those in the team it means the challenge of learning to work together and then maintaining and developing the relationships, but also of giving away decision making power, for patients were to be encouraged to make their own choices. As Lamerton described it 'the doctor's ivory tower is crumbling'. Nurses too are required to make adjustments, as they share their expertise with the patient and their family, and at times to give up a jurisdiction over the physical care and control of in-patients which had previously been solely theirs.

The implementation of the considerable challenges offered by 'family' and 'teamwork' can be considered by looking at different hospice services, for both terms have become subject to different interpretations for all manner of personal, organisational, political, geographical and resource reasons. How nurses on one in-patient unit used the terms is considered here.

NURSES APPLICATION

There was no definitive application of either 'family' or 'team', for although they were useful as principles, the terms were adapted by the staff for use in different circumstances. The patterns of usage though indicate how the nurses approached their work. 'Teamwork' and the 'family' were used in three ways. Firstly, to negotiate roles, secondly to limit the parameters of care and thirdly to organise 'work'. They were not interchangeable and were invoked at different times to explain and reflect upon events.

The team

Within the collective effort to bring about a peaceful death, individual nurses made separate contributions, but it was the whole effect which was discussed and judged in the assessment of patient care. If the nursing team was not working well together, the whole 'family' unit including the patients, were affected because time and commitment were diverted away from patient care to the organisation:

'I think we've managed pretty well, and all the credit's due to the whole team. Because the whole thing about here is team work. Everyone is so important, and if there's a breakdown in teamwork, there's a breakdown in the unit.'

'Teamwork' has to be developed and maintained. It takes planning and organisation to develop a singleness of purpose and to learn to work in an interdisciplinary way. If several nurses left at once the 'team' ethos was threatened and so was the continuity of Byresfold's ideals:

'There's sometimes upsets with the patients, but very seldom upsets with the staff. But I do find that when we do have a lot of new staff, coming at different times, like now, I find that takes a bit of time, until everybody gets to know each other.'

'Team working' was used to explain to outsiders how the staff were able to break down 'normal' hierarchical roles. One means of ensuring the continuity of purpose was to arrange for new staff to be 'paired' with a nurse who was familiar with Byresfold, so that a new, trained nurse would often work with an auxiliary as her teacher. Despite this breaking down of parts of the traditional role structure, traditional work allocation was used to organise the tasks and routines of the unit. As in hospital wards, the sluice was the province of auxiliary nurses, and the treatment room that of the trained staff. Designating responsibility for the running of the unit to the most senior nurses usually worked well, but because nurse hierarchies were used to arrange the work it became a source of disaffection when there was a change in nursing staff:

'I was the first full time staff nurse to come and at the time there was a young enrolled nurse who was very resentful. And I can quite under-

stand. Because the responsibility had been lifted off her and she was put
back to ordinary tasks, without anything. She wasn't given the responsibility. But when they're needed we use them again ... the likes of Margo,
as SEN in the next few weeks is going to be required to do a lot of things
with all the staff nurses leaving. And then the new staff are going to come
in and she too is going to return back to a different level.'

The weekly conference of the 4 doctors, Sister, the district nurse, the
health visitor and the social worker showed the outward commitment to the
value of inter-disciplinary teamwork, with Sister as the representative of
in-patient nurses. On the whole though, auxiliaries had little contact with
the medical staff and even less with the other 'team' members. Under stress,
despite the attempt to overcome the rigidity of 'normal' hierarchies, nurses
would use these same hierarchies as a means of limiting what was expected of
them:

'Jo said to me, "there's a new staff nurse coming so you can show her
what to do". I said, "Jo, I'm only an auxiliary and she's a staff nurse.
I'm doing no extra work telling staff nurses what to do". She said, "oh
you're taking all the wrong attitude now".

The nurses at Byresfold therefore used the hospice principle of teamwork to contrast their approach with 'normal' hospital working but also
invoked traditional ways of dividing work by seniority and training under
particular circumstances. Although this example is intra-disciplinary, it
might usefully be extended to consider how the principle of 'teamwork'
evolves on an inter-disciplinary level.

The family

Constant references to the value of all the staff, and in particular
references to it being a 'family unit' attested to the principle that all
team members have an important contribution to make. As an introduction to
new staff, 'family' with its connotations of warmth and unity was used to
explain the ways the nurses felt about and valued each other and was used in
contrast to the more fleeting commitment in hospitals. It was also a recognition that the patients were part of the morale and atmosphere of the unit.
The term was used loosely, sometimes meaning only the nursing staff, sometimes the ill-people, but more usually to mean both the nurses and the ill-
people:

'Well, I really do feel that this has to be like a family unit. And
we've all got to get on well, and there has to be somebody at the head of
the family. And I think one of the main parts I do, apart from watching over
all the patients is watching over all the staff.'

The reference to 'the family' emphasised the protectiveness which
families offer to each other, but also highlighted the connections rather
than the differences between staff and patients. 'Family' was used to
explain that, as with any family there were ups and downs and disagreements
but that fundamentally everyone cared and looked after each other. New
nurses who did not or could not fit into this system left quickly having
never settled, but those that stayed (the majority), became one of the family.
Thus 'family' was used as a category for including certain people, but by
default then also became an exclusive category ensuring that some people
could not join.

Where the younger nurses looked out for each other like the rest of the
staff, it was the married, older staff, who excelled in giving 'family' care:

'The part-timers that have been here since the beginning are marvellous. They are all married ladies. They do a wonderful day's work, and they're marvellous with the young staff, and marvellous with the patients.'

Use of 'the family' held benefits both in terms of the nursing care of the patients and the inclusion of families, and the well being of the nurses. It served a unifying function. It was also a practical means of making sure that the carers were also cared for, encouraging a free exchange of information, and easy access to each other despite the differences in grades and responsibilities.

One problem with using the analogy of the family was to know its limitations, and to be able to negotiate round expectations that did not fit in with ideas of a family. Although 'family' was used to describe the congenial relations with the patients it was not often used when a patient 'rubbed a nurse up the wrong way'. The balance between the closeness of 'family' and a respectful distance from ill-people and their relatives was sometimes hard to achieve though all the nurses used the analogy of what they would feel like if this were happening to one of their family as a guide to their actions:

'When the niece's father came in I spoke to him, because he came from the same street as my grandfather - and that's how I started the talking. Very distressed, but took a cup of tea and a had a wee blether. And my father is a cancer patient see, and I can always say, "I know what you're going through". I possibly do understand what they're going through because I sometimes think .. oh golly .. how long?'

This empathy was considered by some of the nurses to be less effective, to the point of being rude, when it came to calling some of the older women 'granny'. The use of affectionate terms caused the same kinds of disagreements over the appropriate kind of familiarity with the patients. As Gamarnikow (1978) and Hearn (1982) have highlighted, there is a tendency for medicine to reproduce the social relations of the family, so that father/ mother/child becomes doctor/nurse/patient, with the patient inappropriately taking on the role of child. 'Tootie' is a local term of affection, usually used for small children:

'I think there are basically two kinds of nurses, the Florence Nightingale, mopping the fevered brow, and the cheerer uppers. And I'm mainly the latter. I can do the other when I need to, but this "how are you tonight, tootie?" drives me mad. Especially if I was a patient, I'd hate it.'

Sometimes the familiarity worked in reverse, with a patient identifying a particular nurse with one of her or his family, and this too could cause distress if the nurse felt she had failed the patient in some way:

'Mrs Tomason, that was in the corner bed - she scared the living daylights out of me. She was great big, and what a hoarse voice she had, and she used to call me Maureen .. I looked like her grand-daughter. And it was just when she was dying, and I was doing her with Chris, and she says, "oh, Maureen". and ken, I felt terrible. Because she thought I was her grand-daughter. And you want to be a help, but you canna.'

The sense of 'family' allowed for demonstration of emotions which are uncommon in nursing care. Sorrow, laughter and anger could all be expressed, and importantly tolerated between nurses, and between nurses and patients. The 'rows' that nurses had with one of the patients were a measure of the depth of the relationship rather than its shallowness.

At Byresfold Continuing Care Unit the nurses combined their personal ('family') and professional ('team') experiences as a means of enhancing their care of the dying. Their roles were evolved through a system of 'teamwork' within a 'family unit'. By linking their 'work', that is their timetabled tasks and routines with their approach to 'total patient care', the tensions between 'a family' and 'a team' can be seen as a tension between a form of 'care' which is usually associated with the privacy of the domestic domain, and the organisational requirements of 'work' where inter- and intra-disciplinary hierarchical relationships dictate who does what, where and how. As a result of this there are now some structural difficulties in implementing 'family care' in what, inevitably, remains a place of work:

- family care in the domestic domain remains unclear, and yet with organisations, staff are accountable for their work and how they use their time.

- teams exist to achieve certain pre-arranged outcomes, whereas families have an unspecified remit.

- families are about long term roles with relatively small numbers of people, whereas teams are generally used to deal in the short term with relatively large numbers of people.

- families are private bodies in the sense that their negotiations and communications are amongst a limited number of people. In an in-patient unit, no matter how caring, the sheer number of people involved as patients and staff, in daily contact, alters the type of communication possible.

The list of these contrasts could be developed at length. The purpose of pointing them out is not to imply that the quality of holistic health care cannot or has not improved, but that there are structural obstacles to be negotiated in order to apply the principles. The two frameworks juxtapose a 'family' type of care within a place of work - a highly sophisticated and powerful organisation which health care professionals are trained to conform with.

On a broader perspective there are challenges relevant to all those involved in hospice care, which can be considered using the two frameworks of 'family' and 'team'. Three of these are:

1) how far do we encourage patients and their families to play an active part in decisions about their life and death?

2) how can 'teams' be organised and maintained to sustain 'family' care?

3) how can these changes be accommodated within traditional health care organisation?

As hospice ideas are brought into mainstream health services, the bureaucratic organisational factors which gave rise to impersonal death will affect the way the principles are implemented (Kastenbaum, 1982; James, 1986; Abel, 1986). Modern hospices developed their strategies buoyed up internally by enthusiastic supporters and carefully chosen staff. As the hospice movement matures they are having to learn how to maintain and develop the enthusiasm with new and different staff. Public service hospitals which adopt hospice principles will interpret the principles relative to their own circumstances, and, as each hospice service has, will make their own practical adaptions. 'Family' and 'team' can be a litmus test of how effectively the principles are being implemented. There is inevitable, often creative, tension between the two frameworks, but should a 'team' become merely the tool of the organisation, or 'the family' an inward looking, exclusive unit, it may be time to consider whether the adaption of the hospice principles has become maladaptive.

REFERENCES

Abel, E., 1986, The hospice movement: institutionalising innovation, International Journal of Health Services, 16:71–85.

Gamarnikow, E., 1978, The sexual division of labour: the case of nursing, in: Feminism and Materialism , A. M. Wolpe and A. Kuhn, eds., Routledge and Keegan Paul, London.

Hadlock, D., 1983, Physician roles in hospice care, in Hospice Care: Principles and Practice, C. Corr and D. Corr, eds., Faber and Faber, London.

Hearn, J., 1982, Notes on partriarcy, professionalisation and the semi-professions, Sociology 16:184–202.

James, V., 1986, Care and work in nursing the dying, unpublished PhD thesis, University of Aberdeen.

Kastenbaum, R., 1982, Fantasies in the death system, Death Education, Vol 6:2.

Lack, S., 1983, The hospice concept: the adult with advanced cancer, in Hospice Care: Principles and Practice, C. Corr and D. Corr, eds., Faber and Faber, London.

Lamerton, R., 1973, Care of the dying, Priory Press, Sussex.

Parkes, C. M., 1978, Psychological aspects, in 'The Management of Terminal Disease', C. Saunders, ed., Edward Arnold, London.

Twycross, R., 1973, A plea for eu-thanatos, Prize winning essay of Voluntary Euthanasia Society.

Saunders, C., 1976, What is St. Christopher's? – St. Christophers Annual Report 1976–1977, London.

BEREAVEMENT SUPPORT – THE RELATIONSHIP BETWEEN PROFESSIONALS AND VOLUNTEERS

Marilyn Relf and Ann Couldrick

Sir Michael Sobell House
Churchill Hospital
Oxford, U.K.

Sir Michael Sobell House

Sir Michael Sobell House is an NHS palliative care unit, or hospice, attached to a district general hospital, the Churchill, in Oxford. It is a purpose built hospice and has been open for 10 years. It consists of a 20 bedded inpatient facility, a day centre, and a study centre. In addition it is the base for four Macmillan nurses (or Community Liaison Sisters as they are known in Oxford).

The Bereavement Support Service

Hospices have always sought to provide support to families during the patient's illness and after the patient's death. Our experience of individual work with the bereaved and from holding evening meetings for bereaved relatives and friends led us to decide that a more structured way of offering support was necessary and that this should be provided by volunteers. Grief is not an illness and the use of volunteers, rather than professionals, emphasizes the normality of grief work and makes the relationship between the bereaved and his or her supporters much more equal. At Sobell House, bereavement support is provided in the main by volunteers. The Macmillan Nurses may give support to a small number of families. Inpatient nurses and Day Unit staff have their main contact with the bereaved immediately after the death of a patient.

The Volunteer Service was set up by myself in my then role as Voluntary Services Co-ordinator and by Ann Couldrick who was a Macmillan Nurse and is now the Clinical Nurse Manager at Sobell House. We continue to jointly co-ordinate and supervise the work of the volunteers. We started to select our first volunteers in 1984 and obtained research funds from the Cancer Research Campaign to enable us to evaluate their work in 1986.

Briefly volunteers are carefully selected, attend a training course (45 hours) and attend a fortnightly supervision group. They commit themselves to 16 hours a month and have, on average, five or six clients at a time. In the first two years of the project we had 110 referrals but this is a low figure as this was a time when our first two groups of volunteers were inexperienced and building up their case loads. Between December 1986 and April 1987 we had 41 referrals alone, which is double the previous rate.

Evaluation

As part of our evaluation of the volunteer Service, we decided to examine the attitudes of nurses, doctors and other professional members of the multi-disciplinary team at Sobell House towards the volunteers. We circulated a questionnaire to 35 members of staff and received 24 completed forms back from 14 nurses, 4 Macmillan nurses, 3 doctors and 3 'others' - the physio and occupational therapists and volunteer co-ordinator. We elicited information on staff attitudes about the need for support after bereavement, their knowledge of the volunteer bereavement support service, the referral system and their own training on bereavement.

Background

It has always been difficult for professionals and volunteers to work together. The history of volunteering in Great Britain is rooted in Victorian philanthropy and has produced a stereotype of the volunteer as a female, middle-aged, middle class, 'do-gooder'. However, a recent survey of volunteering (Field and Hedges, 1985) suggested that nearly half the people in Britain are, or have been, involved in some form of volunteer work and that nearly one in five volunteer in any given week. Government spending on volunteering has increased rapidly in the last ten years and the Prime Minister has described volunteering as "the heart of our social welfare provision" and her Government has accordingly targeted a growing variety of programmes and policies towards it. In a climate of unemployment and cuts in public spending, these policies have been met with some hostility and anxiety as well as enthusiasm by the public services and the voluntary sector. It is against this background that along with the Cancer Research Campaign, the Regional Health Authority and District Health Authority is funding our research. Volunteers are now 'allowed' to undertake types of work which would not have been contemplated 15 years ago and the idea of a partnership of professionals and volunteers who work together to provide services is the only way which some services can be developed.

It is not surprising therefore that our survey revealed many contradictions in the professionals' attitudes towards the volunteers.

All the respondents felt that support helps the bereaved to adjust to loss and the majority felt that support would be needed for 18 months. All but five felt that the Bereavement Support Service was an integral part of the work of Sobell House. The five who felt it is an additional service beyond the remit of the Hospice were all in-patient nurses.

Support

The staff felt that support should be offered to those relatives or key carers whom they identified as being 'at risk' rather than to everyone. We asked them who should offer support over and above that available from family/ friends. We gave 6 categories of people who were likely to be thought to have a role in offering support to the bereaved including doctors and clergy. The majority of respondents ticked more than one category with volunteers gaining 22 votes. It would seem, therefore, that Staff are happy to refer key carers to volunteers for follow up in the majority of cases.

When asked who should offer follow-up to key carers who were thought to have more complex problems and be even more 'at risk', volunteers still gained considerable support particularly from the Macmillan Nurses who in the main care for young complex families at home.

The in-patient nurses were more likely to think that psychiatric help would be beneficial or that the clergy or Macmillan Nurses themselves should offer support to the very 'at risk'.

In practice, we have only referred three times to psychiatric services since the project began 2½ years ago, in one case a Consultant in Psychological Medicine shared the intervention with an experienced volunteer. In the second, a local Psychiatric Hospital had to be persuaded to offer sanctuary to a relative who had made two serious suicide attempts. In the third case, a Community Psychiatric Nurse continued her existing involvement with a man after his wife's death.

Clergy too, in practice , have little time to offer support to the bereaved. One survey revealed that clergy conduct a funeral once every nine days and are unlikely to visit the bereaved more than once after the funeral itself (Longbottom 1986).

The staff as a whole think that Macmillan Nurses have an important role to play in supporting the bereaved who are 'at risk' and very 'at risk'. However, the Macmillan Nurses themselves were divided. Two of the four felt that they did not have a role, and felt that their training was inadequate. This is a very interesting and significant contradiction.

Six in-patient nurses felt they should offer support to the bereaved. This is interesting, given that the staff identify that support is necessary for 18 months and it conflicts with the view of eight in-patient nurses who said that they do not have enough time to spend with bereaved relatives around the time of the patient's death anyway. Long term support by in-patient nurses would, therefore, seem impossible without making radical changes to work load and job descriptions.

Anxiety About Volunteers

Although the staff were very much in favour of the volunteer support service, the survey did reveal an underlying anxiety, particularly among in-patient nurses, about the volunteers, who they are and what they are doing. It would seem that the simultaneous introduction of the Volunteer Bereavement Support Service and Primary Nursing as the nursing model at Sobell House have combined to raise awareness of the needs of the bereaved. Primary nursing has given the Staff Nurses much more responsibility – the nurse is aware of the patient's psychological state, knowledge of his/her illness and the relationships in the family in a way that did not happen before the introduction of Primary Nursing. It has, therefore, become much harder for the nurses to see the patient's death as the completion of their task. He/she now recognises that for the family the death is a new beginning.

The nurses want to know how "their" families are getting on after the death but at the same time, admit they would not be able to process information and feed-back on all bereaved relatives. This suggests that the nurse's anxiety reflects their own need to feel that their task has been completed. In discussion they say that they want to know how "their" relatives are getting on. They are ambivalent, however, about hearing that the relatives continue to be distressed.

Macmillan Nurses seem to be more comfortable with the knowledge that volunteers are giving support because they can more realistically acknowledge the length of time that grieving takes and they are aware of their own inability to provide support to more than a few relatives. The needs of the living patient continually push the needs of the bereaved aside and create a growing burden of guilt.

We have looked at many suggestions as to how to remedy the communication gap between the project and the staff and how to give feed-back to fulfill the nurses desire that something is being done without breaking confidentiality or swamping already hard-pressed staff with too much detail. Regular

meetings between staff and volunteers are untenable – the staff and volunteers are too busy. (Staff meetings that we arranged to give feed-back were
so badly attended that they had to be abandoned). Study sessions on the work
of the volunteers and encouragement for staff to seek out the volunteers or
the co-ordinators to find out how people are getting on whom they are particularly worried about, would seem to be a solution and the one we are
currently pursuing.

Training

All the staff (doctors, nurses, Macmillan Nurses and therapists) said
that they would like more training and two-thirds felt inadequately prepared
for their current work with the bereaved. All but one felt they would like
similar training to the volunteers. This training includes counselling
skills and other interpersonal skills as well as training specific to grief
and bereavement. It must be difficult for professionals to see volunteers
taking on work for which they, themselves, feel inadequately prepared.

Moreover, nurses and doctors are trained to expect to make things better
e.g. in the hospice we expect to be able to control pain and symptoms and
the staff are upset and feel inadequate in the few cases where this proves
impossible. Whereas, working with the bereaved, asks the care-giver to help
the client to express his/her pain fully. The bereavement volunteer facili-
tates the expression of emotional pain and does not see the results of his/
her intervention for many months.

It is no wonder that staff sometimes resent the time they spend with
the bereaved and feel that it takes them away from their real work with the
patient. Our culture rewards suffering in silence, being brave, and not
making a fuss. Subliminally, even we, in the hospice share these feelings.

Referral System

Referrals are made by the Primary Nurses and Macmillan Nurses with other
staff adding comments at the weekly psycho-social ward meeting. A referral
form is used which contains a vulnerability questionnaire based on risk
factors identified by Parkes (1975) and Vachon et al.(1982). Unless some
form of objective risk assessment tool is used, decisions are likely to be
made subjectively and judgmentally. The use of the referral form has been
a constant reminder of the needs of the bereaved and has helped the nurses
to understand anticipatory grief and to focus more attention on the key-carer
in the family during the time leading to the death of the patient. By
filling in the forms, the nurses play a vital role in allocating voluntary
resources. Their knowledge and observations are essential and the forms are
filled in after every death. We intend to assess the accuracy of the form
as a predictive tool.

Recommendations

It is essential that volunteer bereavement support services are seen by
staff to be an integral part of hospice care so that referrals can be made
confidently. At Sobell House, we have learnt a great deal from some of the
mistakes we made, the most notable of which was the lack of training available on bereavement for staff. Training volunteers in an area of skill where
professionals feel inadequate can only increase anxiety. From our experience,
we recommend the following:

1. Staff are involved in the planning of support services.
2. Staff are included on the selection and training of volunteers.
3. An objective referral system to identify those 'at risk' is adopted.
    (This is an awareness raising tool itself).

4. Information about the referral system and on the volunteer service be included in all staff orientation programmes including doctors.
5. Volunteers should work in the hospice during the training, preferably in areas where they work alongside inpatient nurses, so that staff and volunteers get to know each other a little, the volunteer feels part of the team and the staff's stereotypes of volunteers are challenged.
6. Training should be available for all staff on interpersonal skills. (We offer staff the opportunity of week-end training sessions with the same trainer as the volunteers).
7. Regular study days on bereavement including case studies based on the volunteers work should be available.

Summary

Staff at Sobell House recognise the importance of bereavement follow-up for those key-carers they identify as being 'at risk'. They can confidently make referrals to volunteers who have been selected and trained to work with the bereaved. Attention should be paid, however, to the staff's own need for training and for information and feedback from the Bereavement Support Service. If gaps in understanding develop, then misconceptions and fantasies will be encouraged and the effectiveness of the support services endangered.

REFERENCES

Field, J. and Hedges B., 1975, A National Survey of Volunteering: Social and Community Planning Research, HMSO. London.

Longbottom, P, 1986, The role of the clergyman in bereavement, Bereavement Care, 5:1.

Parkes, C. M., 1975, Determinants of outcome following bereavement, Omega, 6:303-323.

Vachon, M. L. S., Sheldon, A. R., Lancee, W. J., Lyall, W. A. L., Rogers, J., and Freeman, S. J. J., 1982, Correlates of enduring distress patterns following bereavement: social network, life situation and personality, Psychological Medicine 12:783-788.

THE DEVELOPMENT OF A PROGRAM TO ASSIST SCHOOLAGE CHILDREN IN COPING WITH THE DEATH OF A CLASSMATE

Sharon Frierdich, Andrea Urban, Peggy Possin and
Jan Lehman

University of Wisconsin Hospital and Clinics
Madison, U.S.A.

Cancer remains the leading cause of death in children due to disease in the United States. Approximately 6,400 children are diagnosed with cancer each year. It is a fact, that although the survival rate has increased over the past two decades, approximately one-half of these children will succumb to their disease. Often, children who have failed to respond to treatment may wish to continue to attend school and participate in extra-curricular activities with their peers, as long as physically possible. Most children are aware they are dying and will share this information frankly with their friends and classmates. This information may be viewed as frightening and confusing by their fellow students.

Case Presentation

The impetus for developing a program to assist schoolage children in coping with the death of a classmate, was initiated by the case of Andrea. Andrea was a fun-loving eleven year old girl who had enjoyed several years of intermittent remissions of her brain tumor. She attended school when possible. During her hospitalizations and illnesses at home, her teachers and classmates remained supportive through visits, telephone calls, and cards of well-wishes. Her last aggressive therapy was felt to have left her free of disease. Unfortunately, six months later, Andrea had a recurrence of her tumor. At that time, the pediatric oncology staff informed Andrea and her family that no further treatment options were available. Supportive counsel-ing to assist Andrea, her parents, and sibling cope with Andrea's inevitable death was provided, and a local hospice referral was made to coordinate support and comfort measures in the home.

We failed to ascertain Andrea's intention of returning immediately to school, at which time she informed her classmates that her "tumor was back" and she "was going to die." Tearful and confused students related Andrea's comments to their teacher. The distressed teacher immediately contacted the medical center staff, recounting Andrea's "matter-of-fact" comments and the anxiety this produced in the students. She requested an update on the disease status and suggestions for assisting the school personnel and class-mates in coping with the terminal prognosis. A plan of support was discussed which provided the framework for this program.

This case demonstrates the importance of medical staff in anticipating and adequately preparing the school for the transition of the child, who is terminally ill, back into the classroom. Even if the child is unable to return to school and will die in the home or hospital, we must provide supportive counseling for the often forgotten grievers, the classmates.

Background

A school liaison program between pediatric oncology centers and the school is not a new concept and is an integral component in the standards of care for children with cancer. Contact is made with the school at the time the child is initially diagnosed. Spinetta (1983) reports that this system of communication is essential in providing pertinent and reliable medical facts, dispel myths associated with cancer, i.e. cancer is contagious or inevitably fatal, and prevents inappropriate expectations and psychological euthanasia. Counseling involves helping school personnel come to terms with their own philosophy of life and death, to understand the psychological and physical implications for the child diagnosed with a chronic illness, to appreciate the stress on family members, and to respond to the reactions of the classmates. Often a member of the pediatric oncology team will visit the school to directly provide this information to the students. The theme of this visit at the diagnostic phase is one of hope for cure and optimism for the child's future.

This initial contact with the school helps to develop a relationship with the medical staff, as well as develop a partnership in the delivery of care to the child and family. The continuation of this program is essential when the health status of the child changes, especially during relapses of the disease and the terminal phase of illness. This is critical in re-affirming the role of the educational system for the support of the child and establishment of new goals when appropriate.

Validation for initiation of this program can be found in the litera-ture on death education. Molnar-Stickles (1985) reported that death edu-cation should be viewed as a natural topic for inclusion in the education of schoolage children "because they are not immune to experiencing the death of a loved one, pet, or classmate."

Crase (1984) reports that death education as an educational offering is often controversial and remains a "cultural taboo." Thanatology courses at the elementary level are made available on a sporadic and often loosely-structured basis.

In addition, Leviton (1977) states the importance of formal profession-al preparation for teachers in death education. He stresses the competencies of death educators include not only knowledge of content, but recognition of their own feelings about death, so they can address the topic in a relaxed and supportive style. Today, professional opportunities for educa-tors in death education remain limited and classroom teachers are often inadequately prepared to incorporate this topic into the curriculum, Crase (1980).

It would be advantageous, if prior to a traumatic incident in the school, a structured program in death education was in place, encompassing the elementary years, and expert death educators were available in the school system. When a death of a student is anticipated, counseling could be based on this program. It has been our experience that these prerequi-sites usually do not exist. Homedes and Ahmed (1987) state that health care professionals are in a unique position, due to their knowledge and experience, and can easily be integrated into the educational system in dealing with children and death. Pediatric oncology staff members work with childhood illness and death, and do bereavement counseling as part of their role, consistently addressing these issues with children and their family members. Teachers are usually very receptive to the consultation services from the health care staff. Health care professionals must be willing to share their expertise and become active participants in children's understanding of death, in settings outside the medical facility.

Program Development

The initial step in the development of a structured program assisting classmates in coping with the death of a student was to establish realistic goals. The goals of the program are:

1. Encourage classmates to openly express their fears and concerns about death.

2. Provide information on rituals surrounding death, and death terminology.

3. Provide guidance in interacting with the student who is dying.

4. Provide counselling strategies and resource materials to school personnel and parents of classmates.

5. Develop a support network for the classmates prior and subsequent to the death.

The concept of the support network is to provide several avenues of support and consultation. The participants in this network include the following individuals:

- school personnel   - administrators
                            teacher(s) of child
                            teacher(s) of siblings
                            school nurse
                            health educator
                            school psychologist/social worker
                            religious representative
                            (as in a parochial school)

- medical center staff   - pediatric oncologist
                            primary nurse
                            social worker
                            psychologist/neuropsychologist

- hospice and community   - hospice member
  health services   community health nurse
                            social worker
                            mental health volunteer
                            local physician
                            clergyman (as appropriate)

- child and parent

- parents of classmates

Once the specific members of the support network are identified, we advise planning a strategy meeting. At this meeting the participants are introduced and the roles for implementation of the program are discussed.

Implementation of Program

The program agenda begins as the child enters the terminal phase, and the child and family are made aware of treatment failure. Permission is obtained from the child and family to contact the school and the plan of support for the classmates is outlined. The child and family are given the option of being present during the planning meeting and classroom visit. They may wish to offer suggestions on content to be included. It is advised that preparatory counseling be in place in the school prior to the child's reentry. At this time, counseling is provided to the child about potential reactions of friends and classmates and suggestions given on working through difficult situations.

It is the responsibility of the medical center staff to form the support network, provide initial guidance and resources, and coordinate the implementation of the program.

A referral is made to the local hospice and/or community health care agency, to coordinate home-based care. They are also informed of the school support program and their consent to participate. On several occasions, hospice members, local nurses or physicians have been eager to be involved in the consultation process with the school and have attended and participated in the classroom visit.

The school personnel are contacted and made aware of the change in the child's health status. The child's intention for continued school attendance is shared. The program is described and a time period for the strategy meeting and classroom visit are scheduled. Kilman (1978) states that when a tragedy occurs, children should be informed promptly, prior to the circulation of rumors, and must be given the opportunity to express their feelings in a supportive environment. Information is shared with the teachers about available support services, activities, and resources to help guide the children's expression of feelings, and their usual reactions, based on their developmental stage.

The teacher is encouraged to share with the class, the information of the student's death or impending death. Immediate concerns of the classmates must be addressed, and they are informed that a special period will be arranged to answer their questions. We also encourage the teachers to provide a "question box" in the classroom, to collect the questions and concerns that the children may have. The question box provides a method for "shy" students to express their concerns, as well as allow children to write down their thoughts at impromptu moments. The questions are summarized by the teacher and reviewed by health care staff prior to the classroom visit. In addition, since the classroom visit may stimulate more questions, the question box can be left in place for several weeks, and concerns addressed later.

Since the major support system of children is the family, the teachers are provided with a sample letter to send to the classmates' parents. This letter notifies the parents of the impending death of the student and the potential impact this may have on their child. The letter addresses the interventions by the school with an invitation for parental participation. Parents are also given guidance for home interventions.

The Classroom Visit

In making the classroom visit, over the last nine years, much of what the literature relates, has been borne out through our experience. We attempt to create an environment in which all facets of death are addressed. We begin with a discussion of the disease and its progression, and what happens physically and emotionally during the death process. We relate children's feelings and elicit their responses to information presented, as well as encouraging them to relate their individual experiences. We discuss their thoughts and fantasies, and suggest and encourage problem-solving in developing interventions.

For presentations to all age groups, the use of accurate terminology, visual aids, and a comprehensive bibliography with a sampling of our favorite books, have enhanced the quality of our interaction with the schools. We share also, audio-visual resources, and advise the schools and parents to screen the pertinent materials for content and age appropriateness before their usage. We have come to realize that the more comprehensive the program, utilizing a wide variety of teaching techniques and materials, the better the children's integration of the subject matter. As stated previously, use of the question box, can provide prior insight into what will become the focus of our presentation.

We then begin our discussion describing "what is cancer." We draw "good cells" and "bad cells", we might show an x-ray and/or a doll with a central line catheter. In this way, we are able to address the disease process and why cancer can be so refractory to treatment. Younger children might frequently respond, at this time, relating shots and x-rays they have received, broken bones, cuts and bruises, and relate conversations they have overheard about disease and death. Frequently, this is the only time we curtail the children's exuberance, as it can easily escalate. Older children tend to question the disease process not fully comprehending the frequent absence of a cancer cure.

In the earlier grades (K, 1, and 2), we talk about what death is (one doesn't breathe, eat, move, etc.) We discuss what is real and not real, such as the cartoon characters that are frequently violently abused only to come back next week, or the television actor who is killed off on one show and then returns on another. Children frequently personify death, either as good (an angel) or bad (a headless skeleton), for example. That gives us an opportunity to address the quality of death, using plants and/or animals as examples. How does a dead object look, feel, smell?

We then reiterate that they are healthy and their bodies can recover from illnesses they might contract. We also might address the degree to which one can be sick, and help them to differentiate normal childhood diseases from cancer.

Pre-teens and teenagers may raise questions more explicitly, about how a child might look as he/she is dying, if it is painful, how the body is affected and what feelings coincide with the deterioration of the body during the death process. We become more explicit with terminology in the upper grades, going into more detail about the various types of cancer, specific treatments, and those cancers which are environmental and can be prevented. We differentiate chemotherapeutic drugs from street drugs, and comment on the use of narcotics in pain control.

We talk about the physiologic response of a person close to death, ie. changes in the breathing pattern, bleeding, coma, shortness or rapid breath, and what to do if death occurs while they are present. We discuss other bodily functions and behaviors, ie. emotional withdrawal, decrease in food intake, necessity of transfusions and/or IVs, and the appropriate use of various medications. We might address the susceptibility of the person to other diseases, so that they may not die from cancer, but from something else. Questions are frequently raised about how long the death process takes, when it starts and what makes it end.

During our presentation we encourage questions from the students, teachers, and parents present, as well as requesting their response. Frequently we will relate our experiences at other schools, other children's comments, which enable the students to respond in kind. We inform them that there are no "stupid" questions and model ways to "deal with" difficult situations, ie. "how would you feel if 50 kids came up to you and asked how you were feeling?" What might be a better way of finding out how someone was doing?

We may possibly address how different cultures view death and might speak about religion and how a particular child/family might cope. We stress the absence of how different people deal with a stiutation in different ways, and how to "think" before speaking (as we all can ask offensive questions without realizing it).

We suggest alternate ways of expressing feelings and emotions for each developmental stage. Drawings by the younger children, use of puppets, movement and music can be beneficial in acknowledging those emotions. Fifth and sixth graders, as well as teens can keep a diary and address comments and concerns to parents. We also state that some children may find communication with parents difficult at times, and may turn to another relative, friend, or teacher. Whatever the means of expression, we firmly reiterate that all thoughts and feelings are "normal", and that there is no timetable for grieving. We inform children of all ages that they may carry a death experience with them throughout their lifetime, as well as support each person's individual experience.

As we all know, younger children are quick to discuss their experiences with doctors and nurses. As well as acknowledging the physical experiences of children, we must also address their fantasies. With the younger child, we are quick to dispel their notions that "thoughts kill", or that they, in any way, can cause another's death. We can help them to integrate how their senses react ie., they need not be afraid of the hair and/or weight loss of a dying person. We ask how they would feel if someone would stare at them or laugh?. We address helpful ways in which children can respond to a friend if they visit them at home or in the hospital, or if the child comes to school. What can they say and do, how do they act? We might even discuss the funeral rites, whether or not the body might be displayed and how should they touch their friend, how might the body feel, and what to do if they feel like crying or laugh. Sanctioning those feelings and problem-solving with the children is invaluable as they progress through the experience.

We have already mentioned several interventions utilized in verbally and non-verbally dealing with the subject of death, and now want to further enumerate several of the suggestions that school personnel and students have made. Their remembrances can be as creative as the students, school personnel, and family wish. Examples are:

- Third grade children continued to visit a hospital, the home, and encouraged the dying child to come to school two days before her death. Their cards and pictures filled her room.

- A girl scout troop sang several of a 13 year old's favorite songs at her funeral.

- Children wrote their favorite story/anecdote/poem about a child and presented them to the family.

- A 10 year old's funeral was held in the school he so dearly loved.

- A tree was planted in the school yard in memory of a child.

- A middle school closed two hours early so that students and teachers might attend the funeral.

- A picture and biography were hung in a high school hallway.

- The yearbook and class newsletter were dedicated to the student.

- The picture of the student was pasted to his desk after his death and left vacant and in place the remainder of the school year.

- A plaque immortalized a 12 year old's messy locker.

- A class wrote farewell letters before the child died and then read them at the funeral.

One more important point to make is in addressing the needs of the sibling(s). As you well know, not only have the siblings received less attention during the illness but afterwards the parents may find it difficult to be supportive to their other children. Therefore, we feel, the school can be an invaluable resource in providing an arena in which the sibling can meet with success and find support that may not be available in the home.

We frequently include the sibling's classroom in our presentation and alert his/her teacher(s) to their immediate concerns and those which could erupt years later. We encourage the sibling's involvement with the affected child throughout his/her illness as well as through the death process. The school situation can most positively enhance that adjustment.

Follow-up

Children who are the friends, classmates and sibling(s) of a deceased child are often indirect victims and are subject to emotional turmoil and many fantasies. Kilman, (1978). Therefore, a comprehensive, structured approach to death, in a supportive environment will further enhance their coping abilities throughout life. We must not place a time period on the extent of their grief and we must be open to address their concerns whenever they arise. Families, school personnel, and medical staff need to seek out messages hidden in unusual behavior. It is our responsibility to facilitate the grieving of those children who are having difficulty adjusting, and make available to their families, appropriate resources.

While our only documented follow-up has been word-of-mouth, the program has met with great success, and teachers have informed us that they have noticed the children have appeared more comfortable in discussing and commenting on what happened, and how they felt about the death of their peer.

References

Crase, D., 1980, The health educator as death educator: Professional preparation and quality control. The Journal of School Health, 10:568-571.

Crase, D., 1984, Minimizing resistance to death education, Health Values Achieving High Level Wellness, 8:6.

Homedes, N., and Ahmed, S., 1987, In my opinion...death education for children. CHC, 16:1.

Kilman, A.S., 1978, "Crisis: Psychological First Aid for Recovery and Growth" Holt, Rinehart, and Winston, New York.

Leviton, D., 1977, The role of the schools in providing health education. in: "Death Education: Preparation for Living", B.P. Green, D.P. Irish eds.

Molnar-Stickles, L., 1985, Effect of a Brief Instructional Unit in Death Education on Death Attitudes of Prospective Elementary School Teachers, Journal of School Health, 55:6.

Spinetta, P., Spinetta, J., 1983, The child with cancer returns to school: preparing the teacher. <u>in</u> "The Child and Death", J. Schowalter, P. Patterson, M. Tallmer, A. Kutscher, S. Gullo and D. Peretz, eds, Columbia University Press, New York.

PART THREE

EVALUATION

BATTLE FATIGUE IN HOSPICE/PALLIATIVE CARE

Mary Vachon

Department of Psychiatry and Behavioural Science
University of Toronto
Toronto, Canada

Battle fatigue has been described as "A psychoneurosis occurring among soldiers engaged in active warfare, and often making continued service in danger zones impossible, (Stein, 1969)." From the perspective of a hospice/ palliative care professional, the phenomenon can be viewed as the syndrome which may make it difficult, if not impossible for the worker to continue to perform the functions associated with one's role with dying persons and their families. The concept of "shell shock" to which someone consulting the dictionary regarding battle fatigue is referred is seen to be characterized "variously by loss of self-command, speech, sight, or other powers, formerly believed to be brought on by the shock of exploding shells in battle, but now explained as the result of cumulative emotional and psychological strain of warfare," (Stein, 1969). Both concepts are perhaps somewhat melodramatic to describe the symptoms experienced by those in hospice work. Nevertheless, many may be able to identify with the concept of difficulty with the cumulative exposure to the suffering and deaths of large numbers of patients and to the grief of their family members. For some, this exposure may make continued service in hospice or palliative care units impossible.

The concept of battle fatigue can perhaps best be compared with the popular concept of "burnout" which has been characterized as "The progressive loss of idealism, energy and purpose experienced by people in the helping professions as a result of the conditions of their work" (Edelwich with Brodsky, 1980).

Burnout is generally seen to be the interaction between the needs of a person to sacrifice him/herself for a job and a job situation which places inordinate demands on an individual. In a large study of hospice staff burnout was found to be associated with high educational levels, long tenure and full time status (Mor and Laliberte, 1984). Edelwich and Brodsky (1980) have noted that burnout can occur not only in an individual but also within a system (Vachon, 1986).

The concept of battle fatigue is meant to imply a state which might occur before burnout. As with the treatment of battle fatigue in wartime situations, after an initial period away from the work situation, the best treatment for those suffering from work-related battle fatigue may well be close contact with others in the trenches. Total removal from the stressor such as resignation from one's position may not be the best treatment. Unlike the wartime situation, the professional suffering from battle fatigue may be able to take some time to reflect on the source of stress, consider ways to alleviate some of the stressors and only then take the time to decide whether or not the best decision would be to leave the work situation.

The findings of the present study of stress in hospice/palliative care workers challenges some of those who would suggest that hospice workers are more vulnerable to battle fatigue or burnout than other caregivers to the critically ill, dying and bereaved.

This paper analyzes the problems experienced by multidisciplinary hospice teams using data collected as part of a larger study of the stress experienced by careivers to the critically ill, dying and bereaved in a variety of settings including: obstetrics, pediatrics, oncology, hospice, critical care, emergency rooms, chronic care and bereavement work (Vachon, 1987). The data were gathered internationally and thus the terms hospice and palliative care are used interchangeably, reflecting the different terms used in various countries.

The data gathered show that work stress is by no means exclusive to hospice workers. Perhaps unexpectedly, most of the stressors, caregivers reported, when asked about the stress they experienced in caring for the critically ill and dying were not directly related to work with clients and their families but, rather to difficulties with colleagues and with institutional hierarchies. This article will provide an overview of the sources of stress, its manifestations and coping strategies used by hospice caregivers.

METHOD

Sample

The subjects are part of a larger sample of 581 caregivers from a variety of professional groups, specialty areas and practice settings. They were interviewed in Canada, the United States, Europe, and Australia. The subsample of those in hospice work consisted of 60 interviews involving an international convenience sample of 100 caregivers including: physicians (38%); nurses (42%); social workers (13%); clergy (2%); volunteers (3%); physiotherapists (3%); and others (9%). Three percent of the sample were under 30 years of age; 45% were between 30-45 and 52% were over 45 years of age. Caregivers interviewed about hospice stress were from Canada (63%); United States (13%); Great Britain, Australia and South Africa (22%); and non-English speaking countries (2%).

RESULTS

Work Environment Stressors

It might be assumed that the primary occupational stressors of those working with the critically ill, dying and bereaved would be dealing with dying persons and their families. Such was not the case. It was found that the work-related stressors primarily involved difficulty with the work environment, (48%) and occupational role (29%). Patients and families accounted for a smaller percentage (17%) as did illnesses (7%). The top ten stressors reported were: communication problems with "others" in the system, role ambiguity, team communication problems, communication problems with administration, role conflict, the nature of the system, inadequate resources, unrealistic expectations of the organization, patient/family communication problems and patient/family coping or personality problems. None of the top ten stressors mentioned involved direct difficulty in dealing with dying persons or their family.

Communication problems with "others" in the system often involved
difficulty with other specialties who were seen as either not appreciating
those in hospice or not appropriately referring clients to them. Frequently
this problem evolved from the fact that the other specialties within the
health care system had not been adequately prepared for the development of
the hospice and resented the resources made available to new programmes.
There was sometimes rivalry for patients as caregivers in oncology or chronic
care learned the basic concepts about symptom relief and supportive services
from hospice programmes or seminars and then integrated these concepts into
their own care, rather than referring patients to palliative care programmes.
At times other services were seen as simply "hanging on" to their clients
and "depriving" them of the benefits of a hospice programme.

As hospices became an accepted part of the health care system there were
sometimes problems with continued financing. Programmes which have to
compete for funds sometimes found it difficult to continue to obtain funding
once the programme had become established and was no longer simply an interesting new fad.

Hospice physicians at times found it difficult to maintain credibility
within the medical profession when they were devoting their major medical
efforts to palliative medicine. At times this was seen to be an inferior
type of medical practice. This was particularly a problem in the United
States where there are almost no physicians who have been in full time
medical practice within a hospice setting for a period of ten years. Difficulty in obtaining financial remuneration is part of the problem but there
is also concern that unless a physician is older and prepared to spend the
remainder of a professional life in doing hospice work, one might be in-
advertently limiting one's career possibilities.

There were also interprofessional communication problems which developed.
Hospice programmes were sometimes administered by nurses, social workers,
or administrators who had a major role in deciding who should be admitted
to the programme. For some physicians this was a very real problem as they
felt that they no longer had the control of access to services.

Role ambiguity involved a lack of clear-cut professional role definitions. While one of the major strengths of hospice work is the role blurring
(one group performing roles which another group might traditionally be
expected to do) which may occur, this can also serve as a significant
stressor for those who feel that others are assuming their roles without
their gaining other roles in return. Physicians sometimes feel that nurses
are overextending their traditional professional roles and physicians may
become threatened and concerned when it appears that nurses are almost
practicing medicine without a medical license. This may occur particularly
with nurses involved in home care work who have more freedom to make
independent decisions than do nurses in in-patient programmes.

Social workers and clergy may feel that other professionals are usurping
their roles as nurses are talking about spiritual matters and physicians are
doing family counselling. One social worker expressed considerable frustration when she said "things would be a lot better around here if only the
physicians would stop talking to the families and leave that to the social
workers". The physician presumably was deriving some increased role satisfaction from this expanded role but her new expertise was in turn threatening
the social worker.

It is helpful for hospices to recruit staff members who are sufficiently
experienced within their own profession so as to not be threatened by the
role blurring which occurs within hospice. This is of course the ideal.
Professional turf disputes may well become more common as some hospice

programmes suffering from fiscal restraints are being forced to drop all "non-essential" services. A professional who feels that another person's increasing expertise is in the long term threatening to his or her job may well experience considerable job stress.

There may also be role ambiguity with regard to team leadership issues. In situations in which a physician is not the head of the team there may be difficulty with issues of authority and responsibility especially when the legal issue of responsibility is concerned.

Team communication problems were ranked as being somewhat less of a problem amongst hospice caregivers than they were in other specialty areas. This is probably because of the effort which hospice workers put into team development. It may also be reflective of uniting together against the "others who do not understand us".

Team communication problems have been recognized as a stressor in other studies of stress in hospice by (Mount and Voyer, 1980; Lyall, Rogers and Vachon, 1976; Lyall, Vachon and Rogers, 1980; and Yancik, 1984). Team communication problems involved a lack of recognition of the expertise of others on the team, "incest" within the team, a lack of team stability, interprofessional rivalry and intraprofessional rivalry.

The lack of recognition of the expertise of others often involved a lack of trust in allowing others to have the freedom to perform creatively within the professional or volunteer role. There was sometimes also professional jealousy at the fact that someone else might be performing "my" role as well as or better than I might be able to do. Difficulties with issues of confidentiality could also occur. Team members could become rivalrous with regard to who was able to obtain the most confidential information from patients or who was able to have the "most meaningful" relationships.

Incest on the health care team is not discussed very often in the literature on stress in health care workers but it can be a significant stressor. White (1978) has noted that incest within families often occurs when the family is isolated from the larger community. So too may hospice teams have difficulty with incest when they see themselves as performing just within their limited specialty and not as part of the larger health care system. There may be a turning in upon the group to meet all of ones needs which may include familial and sexual needs. Familial rivalry patterns between staff members who assume the "parent" roles and those who assume the "child" roles may develop. Such role patterns may not always be recognized as such. One young male physician found himself having difficulty in communicating with the middle-aged nurse with whom he worked until he recognized that they were both unconsciously acting out old familial roles with the nurse expecting that he would be "a good boy" and order what she told him to order and his feeling resentful and "pushed around" by this "mother figure".

Sexual liaisons between team members are also not uncommon. In part of course these represent a "celebration of life". However, such liaisons may lead to judgement errors as well as team communication problems.

A lack of team stability often occurred when some staff members left, either because of work stress, team communication problems or for other reasons. The lack of team stability was particularly problematic for teams which had considerable turnover (Yancik a), reflecting chronic team stress, as well as for teams which had considerable team stability until one or more key team members left. Sometimes a domino effect was created with the fact that a key person or key people left, leading others to question why they were staying and gaining the courage to leave. Other times the others "stayed behind" feeling resentful and abandoned and finding it very difficult to integrate others into the team, thereby creating a situation in which the newcomers were apt to leave after only a short time. This type of situation often led to reflections about the "good old days" when there was plenty of money for hospice care, more personal gratification and team spirit.

Intergroup rivalry within palliative care teams took place amongst those of different disciplines and often reflected concern about one's place on the team. One physician mentioned that he had difficulty relating to other disciplines on a horizontal plane and felt guilty because he could not clearly identify his contribution on the team. He was aware that he often felt defensive when other team members made suggestions to him. At these times he tended to feel criticized, disorganized and inadequate. He acknowledged feeling this way because others thought of things he hadn't. At these times interactions often led to anger and conflict on the team rather than being dealt with openly and non-aggressively. In other teams such conflicts sometimes led to obstructing the work of others or withdrawing from the team (Vachon, in press).

Hospice teams have particular difficulty in handling anger and conflict. Such conflicts may involve power struggles amongst various disciplines dealing with issues such as credit for the programme and control over the services offered. Handling such conflict within a hospice team is difficult. A social worker at one prominent hospice observed that "there is more conflict here than at almost any other general hospital". An important team issue becomes how staff can express anger in the calm of a hospice (Vachon, in press).

Intraprofessional rivalry occurred when members of the same discipline had difficulty in dealing with one another. Sometimes this occurred between factions of new and old guard caregivers. The "old guard" would make it clear that they did not feel that the "new guard" had the same philosophy or provided to the same level of care which had previously been available. In the United States some of these conflicts occur when patients come into home care hospice programmes while still utilizing many technological devices such as venous implant devices or TPN. The "old guard" may not be used to dealing with technology and may be threatened. Rather than acknowledging their discomfort, there may be power struggles within the team as each group struggles to show that it has an important role to play.

Communication problems with administration often involved the feeling that the hospice programme was not receiving sufficient recognition within the larger hospital system if the programme was part of a larger system. Within free standing hospices there was sometimes the feeling that the new generation of hospice administrators, who may be trained as administrators and not as clinicians, do not really understand what the front line workers are trying to accomplish. There may be resentment of administrators who want staff to be aware that the programme needs to be cost-effective in order to survive.

In other hospice programmes there seemed to have been insufficient forethought prior to the development of the programme as to the long term costs of a high staff-patient/family ratio, good medical coverage, support systems for staff and bereavement services, all of which may be costly to maintain in the long term. Over time, palliative care unit staff may find that they have difficulty getting the staff they feel they need to continue to provide their services. This may either be because caregivers are no longer interested in applying to hospices for employment or else the staff may feel that administration encourages highly qualified applicants to work in other services.

Role conflict has been defined as the extend to which expectations for the roles one performs are compatible or in conflict (Fry, Lech and Rubin, 1974). Role conflict may occur within one's professional role when an individual holds more than one role simultaneously and the demands of one role may conflict with the demands of another (interrole conflict) (Schmalenberg and Kramer, 1979). For example, a nurse may feel in conflict as to her role as a team member who should uphold what the physician says and her role as a patient advocate. Role conflict may also occur because as one operates in more than one role, more than one group of people may have expectations of how one should perform (intrarole conflict). For example, a social worker may be aware that there are limited resources which can be offered by the hospice programme in which she works; yet she may feel pressured by a patient and family member needs to provide more than the services which are available.

Finally, role conflict may occur when the expectations of a role are in opposition to one's personality characteristics or needs (self-role conflict). Caregivers who were initially attracted to hospice because they felt it provided the ideal care for dying people may feel quite conflicted when they feel that they are no longer able to offer the ideal such service.

The nature of the system or institution may be a stressor for those who feel that in hospice no matter how hard one works the outcome will always be the same - the person will die. While some caregivers receive significant role gratification from helping to ease the suffering which may accompany death and bereavement; others find that there is too much stress generated for them from the constant exposure to loss, death and grief experiences (Millet, 1983). In part this is the result of person-environment fit difficulties (French, Rodgers and Cobb, 1974). Caregivers come into hospice with different needs and expectations of the organization and the organization has different expectations of the caregiver. When these needs and expectations do not mesh or when they change over time, one may experience person environment misfit (Vachon, 1985). Such misfit may well occur with caregivers who tire of constant exposure to death and need to see at least some people improve.

Mount and Voyer (1980) have documented other stressors within the work environment including responsibility without power, duties outside traditional nursing roles and heavy physical care demands.

Inadequate resources include a lack of financial resources to provide for a variety of services as well as a lack of staff and volunteers to provide the services required.

Unrealistic expectations of the organization often involved unrealistic expectations of the amount of time staff could be expected to contribute to the programme. While many hospices began as volunteer programmes, it is usually difficult to continue a programme with volunteer help alone. Organizations often expect caregivers to spend a considerable amount of off-duty time in a voluntary capacity in order to meet patient needs.

This constant being "on call" generally does not work well over a period of many years.

Patient/family communication problems occurred when patients were confused, generally as a result of their illness. Particular problems were experienced with patients who had brain tumours and were no longer able to communicate with staff. As the rewards from caregiving decreased and patients simply required heavy physical care, the staff often had difficulty. Some units solved this problem by limiting the number of patients with brain tumours they would admit to their unit. Others solved the problem by limiting the amount of time they would allow patients with brain tumours to stay on a palliative care unit. One woman spoke of being pleased to have her husband admitted to a palliative care home care programme when he was diagnosed as having a brain tumour and she was told that he had only a few weeks to live. When he was still alive and completely immobile two years later he was admitted to a palliative care unit but she was told that he would have to leave after six weeks if he did not die within that time frame. Needless to say, this caused the wife considerable distress, although it might have served to decrease staff distress.

Other caregivers reported stress from caring for patients with different religious beliefs or a different value system from that of the caregiver. Often caregivers did not know how to respond to the needs of these patients and families, felt guilty and in response distanced from the clients. Communication problems could also occur when the patient/family were of a similar background to that of the caregiver. Staff could feel threatened and respond in inappropriate ways.

Patient/family coping or personality problems involved patients and family members who did not respond to the illness or death experience in the way caregivers might expect. This included patients and families who might have been significantly depressed, angry, withdrawn, psychotic, denied their illness or impending death, acted out with drugs or alcohol or used avoidance behaviour to deal with the illness/death experience. Staff members also had difficulty in dealing with multiproblem families wherein the illness and impending death only complicated pre-existing problems. While it was difficult to handle such problems in the in-patient hospice setting it became even more difficult when the patient was being cared for at home. Staff members spoke of having to deal with violent family members, especially adult sons and husbands whose response to the impending death was one of panic which was dealt with through drinking leading to violent behaviour. While staff members felt sorry for the patients in this situation and wished they could be more helpful, the staff eventually had to decide that these clients had chosen to live with this situation for many years and it was not always going to be possible to intervene and resolve the problem.

In these situations the family members often had difficulty in "letting go". When patients and families were not at the same point with regard to "letting go", problems often occurred (Barstow, 1980, Gotay, Crockett and West, 1985 and Vachon, in press).

MANIFESTATIONS OF STRESS

The major manifestations of stress in hospice caregivers were staff conflict, feelings of depression, grief and guilt; job/home interaction and feelings of helplessness. In earlier work by the author and her colleagues, it was found that over half the palliative care staff surveyed on one unit had stress scores almost twice as high as those of newly widowed women and higher than those of women newly diagnosed as having breast cancer (Lyall, Rogers, & Vachon, 1976; Lyall, Vachon, & Rogers, 1980; Vachon, et al 1981-2; Vachon et al 1982). In addition, these nurses were more apt to report psychophysiological symptoms such as sleep disturbances, loss of energy and nervousness, than were nurses on other units. Over time their stress decreased and was comparable to that experienced by nurses on another new unit in the same hospital (Vachon, in press). (Chiriboga, Jenkins and Bailey, (1983) also studied hospice nurses and found that those who did not initially admit to finding hospice work difficult, had more stress in the long term.

Staff conflict was evidenced in scapegoating, rivalry, power struggles, displaced hostility and separation anxiety. The scapegoating often reflected problems in team dynamics. Edelwich and Brodsky (1980) suggest that in teams which are in the process of burning out there are often antagonistic pairings – two or more people team up to complain about the others. In some situations all of the problems which exist within the team are displaced onto one team member who becomes the scapegoat. Some teams seem able to function only when there is a clearly identified scapegoat. When that person leaves, the team will often unconsciously restructure and identify another scapegoat. It appears in such situations that the team is able to displace much of their work anxiety and feelings of impotence in this way.

Rivalry and power struggles have been discussed in the section on stressors. In that situation they have become a chronic problem. As a manifestation of stress, rivalry and power struggles may be of a shorter duration and as such occur primarily when staff members are under stress because of work environment problems, often having to do with a feeling that their role is being threatened or not being recognized.

Displaced hostility occurs when caregivers who are angry about one issue express their anger about a different issue. For example a caregiver who is angry that a patient died and "abandoned her" may displace this anger onto the hospice administrator for not providing sufficient staff coverage to have allowed her to stay with that person as he died.

When caregivers leave the work situation, for whatever reason, there may be considerable separation anxiety on the part of colleagues who become angry at the person for choosing to leave and "abandon us"., Underlying this manifestation of stress is the primitive belief that patients may die and "abandon" us because they cannot help it but our colleagues must not choose to leave and must not feel that they are going on to something better.

Feelings of depression, grief and guilt – caregivers are prone to feelings of depression and grief in response to the death of patients. However, not all depression and grief evolves from death. Caregivers also grieve in response to other losses which may include the loss of support from colleagues as well as the loss of self esteem which may evolve from not performing as well as one might have liked to in one's professional role (see also Weisman, 1981) or from a lack of support from one's colleagues. Caregivers who are very invested in their professional role and lack outside validation of their self worth may be particularly vulnerable to feelings of grief and depression.

Freud (1963) has distinguished mourning from melancholia-grief from depression, by the fact that the latter involves a loss of self-esteem which is not commonly seen in grief. Caregivers who find themselves suffering from a low sense of self-esteem and feelings of worthlessness, especially if these symptoms are accompanied by the other symptoms of depression such as sleep disturbances, weight changes, loss of libido and constipation would do well to seek professional help.

Caregiver grief and depression, with or without feelings of guilt, may be acute and follow immediately upon a loss or such emotions may be chronic and evolve over a considerable period of time in response to repeated losses. It is also relevant to note that not only may individuals suffer from chronic grief, so too may their teams which need to evolve healthy mechanisms for grieving for the losses which they have sustained.

Job/home interaction increased with age and was more likely to be reported in the study as a whole by men rather than by women. In hospice work, caregivers were often on call while at home which could seriously interfere with home life. In addition, some seemed to be psychologically involved with their patients for much of the time they were at home. One wife of a hospice physician said that she wished that just once she could feel that as her husband made love to her, he was concentrating just on her instead of on all of his dying patients. Female caregivers reported that their husbands insisted that books on death should not be kept on their bedside tables if they were going to join them in bed.

It is also interesting to speculate on the effect this type of work has on the children of caregivers. One minister said that when he called his young daughter to dinner one night she whispered back that she could not come because one of her dolls was dying and she could not leave her alone. This exposure to death may be quite healthy for children or it may result in later difficulties – only time will tell.

Feelings of helplessness and insecurity arise in part because of caregiver's unrealistic expectations of themselves (Vachon, 1979). It is not always possible to have the complete alleviation of all symptoms, psychosocial problems and spiritual crises before the time of death as well as a smooth course of bereavement after the death (Vachon, in press).

COPING WITH HOSPICE/PALLIATIVE CARE STRESS

As is the case with battle fatigue in wartime situations, the most effective antidote for the alleviation and prevention of stress within the hospice setting had to do with a sense of team philosophy, team support and team building. Hospice workers also reported using the coping mechanisms of a sense of competence, control and pleasure in one's work; developing control over one's clinical practice; having a personal philosophy of illness, death and one's professional role as well as obtaining increased education as being effective coping mechanisms. Only the first of these coping mechanisms will be discussed in the present paper as it is the most important for the concept of battle fatigue. The reader who is interested in a more thorough discussion of the concepts is referred to the author's larger study (Vachon, 1987). In general, hospice workers reported fewer stressors, fewer manifestations of stress and more coping mechanisms than any of the other professional groups surveyed (Vachon, 1986).

Team philosophy, team support and team building was the most commonly mentioned coping mechanism in hospice caregivers and was more apt to be mentioned by experienced caregivers (those in the age groups 30–45 and over 45).

Often hospice staff members had gone through great efforts to work on team building. Generally, but not always, they had a sense of team philosophy and they at least paid some lip service to the concept of responsibility for supporting one another. It was, however, generally recognized that caregivers could not expect to receive all of their support from their colleagues.

A team philosophy is sometimes clearly articulated, understood and followed by all team members. At other times it is not clearly formulated but exists primarily in the mind of the team leader. A team philosophy generally consists of a set of norms, or the unwritten rules that govern a group. "When they are understood as such, or just 'felt', they are powerful determinants of how team members behave. They constitute 'the way we do things around here' " (Mount and Voyer, 1980, p.465).

At one internationally recognized hospice the general philosophy was, "We don't try to be the perfect hospice, but we have the notion of being a

'good enough hospice' which allows people to have a 'good enough death'."
This type of philosophy can keep staff members from suffering inappropriately
when patients do not die in the "ideal way". It allows staff to be open to
constant learning without having the unrealistic expectation that everything
will be perfect (Vachon, 1987).

An effective hospice philosophy integrates a clear understanding of the
roles and expectations of team members and usually recognizes and allows for
the overlapping of roles. Mount and Voyer (1980) comment that in a successful hospice, it is necessary for each member of the team caring for patients
to know what all the other involved team members are doing and why they are
doing it. This is crucial to a philosophy of sharing information rather
than hoarding it to oneself and attempting to have individual "special"
relationships with patients. Doyle (1982) comments that good terminal care
demands role overlap and a mutual appreciation and support of one another's
role that can be so difficult that some caregivers will find themselves
unable to work in this kind of setting because their own personal insecurity
may become evident to them (Vachon, 1987).

An effective team philosophy also allows for time to grieve for the
deaths and losses that caregivers experience through the use of death rounds
(Vachon, 1987), attendance at funeral services or the integration of some
type of memorial service into the hospice programme.

Team building implies the development of skills which a team member will
need in order to function as a member of this particular team. It is pre-
supposed that an individual team member comes with a reasonable number of
skills of their own professional discipline before beginning work on any
multidisciplinary team. It is only after one has developed the skills of
one's own profession that it is possible to become members of a team in
which the expectation involves considerable role blurring (Vachon, 1987).

Team support serves to buffer group members from battle fatigue and as
well can serve to help those who suffer from the syndrome. Social support
is a function of a team which evolves over time and is probably most
effective only after the team members are secure in themselves and are able
to reach out and trust one another. While new teams will start by having
a firm commitment to a philosophy of team support, it takes a considerable
amount of time before that philosophy can become a reality and before team
members are really able to reach out and meet the needs of other people on
the team (Vachon, 1987). It must be noted that it is difficult for some
teams to provide support for colleagues whose approach or personality differs
from that of other group members. In addition there may be great difficulty
in a team in providing support for a team member who may be trying to decide
whether or not to leave the team (Vachon, in press, b).

Support for colleagues implies a certain level of reciprocity which is
sometimes lacking in teams. Some caregivers can only support, others can
only take, while still others feel that one should be able to take care of
one's own needs for support. While the ideal would be to assume that teams
would reach out to a colleague experiencing battle fatigue, the reality
sometimes is that the team may become threatened and withdraw from those in
need of help.

Team support mechanisms must function at both the formal as well as
informal levels. The former might involve regular team support meetings,
rounds, informal social occasions as well as retreats, while the latter
involves being accessible to colleagues in need, even when one might find
the need to be personally threatening. It must be noted, however, that
hospice teams do exist primarily to care for patients and family members.
When team support assumes a role which almost threatens the real purpose

of the team, then it is necessary to reassess priorities. Teams may well need to develop support mechanisms which recognize that it is possible to meet many, but not all the needs of team members. An effectively functioning team can identify the fact that some needs may require additional outside resources and will make provision for these to be available as necessary.

In conclusion, I have identified the ten major sources of stress reported by a group of 100 hospice/palliative care caregivers representing a variety of professional groups, clinical settings and countries of practice. Battle fatigue is seen to be one possible outcome of occupational stress and involves feelings of depression, grief and guilt, staff conflict, job/home interaction and feelings of helplessness and impotence. A sense of team philosophy, team support and team building can be instrumental in preventing, alleviating and curing battle fatigue.

REFERENCES

Barstow, J., 1980, Stress variance in hospice nursing, Nursing Outlook, 28(12):751-754.
Chiriboga, D. A., Jenkins, G. and Bailey, J., 1983, Stress and coping among hospice nurses: Test of an analytic model, Nursing Research, 32:294-299.
Doyle, D., 1982, Nursing education in terminal care, Nurse Education Today, 2:4-6.
Edelwich, J., and Brodsky, A., 1980, "Burn-out Stages of Disillusionment in the Helping Professions", Springer, New York.
French, J. R. P., Rodgers, W. and Cobb, S., 1974, Adjustment as person-environment fit, in "Coping and Adaption", G. Coelho, D Hamburg and J. Adams, eds., Basic Books, New York.
Freud, S., 1963, Mourning and melancholia, in "General Psychological Theory", Collier Books, New York.
Fry, R. E., Lech, B. A., and Rubin, I., 1974, Working with the primary care team: The first intervention, in "Making Health Care Teams Work" H. Wise, R. Beckhard, I Rubin and A.L. Kyte, eds., Ballinger, Cambridge, Mass.
Gotay, C. C., Crocket, S., and West, C., 1985, Palliative home care nursing: Nurses' perceptions of roles and stress, Canada's Mental Health, 33(2):6-9.
Lyall, W. A. L., Rogers, J., and Vachon, M. L. S., 1976, Professional stress in the care of the dying, Palliative Care Service Report, Royal Victoria Hospital, Montreal.
Lyall, W. A. L., Vachon, M. L. S., and Rogers, J., 1980, A study of the degree of stress experienced by professionals caring for dying patients, in "The Royal Victoria Hospital Manual on Palliative/Hospice Care: A Resource Book", I. Ajemian and B. Mount, eds., ARNO Press, New York.
Millet, N., 1983, Hospice: A new horizon for social work, in "Hospice Care, Principles and Practice", C.A. Corr and D.M. Corr, eds., Springer, New York.
Mor, V., and Laliberte, L., 1984, Burnout among hospice staff, Health and Social Work, 9(4)274-283.
Mount, B., and Voyer, J., 1980, Staff stress in palliative/hospice care, in "The RVH Manual on Palliative/Hospice Care", I. Ajemian and B. Mount, eds., The Free Press, New York.
Schmalenberg, C., and Kramer, M., 1979, "Coping with Reality Shock, The Voices of Experience", MA: Nursing Resources Inc., Wakefield.
Stein, J., (Editor in Chief), 1969, "The Random House Dictionary of the English Language", Random House, New York.
Vachon, M. L. S., 1979, Staff stress in the care of the terminally ill, Quality Review Bulletin 5:13-17.

Vachon, M. L. S., 1987, "Occupational Stress in the Care of the Critically Ill, Dying and Bereaved", Hemisphere, New York.

Vachon, M. L. S., (in press-a), Team stress in palliative/hospice care, The Hospice Journal.

Vachon, M. L. S., (in press-b), Personality and lifestyle of hospice caregivers, in "Proceedings of the 1986 National Conference on Hospice Management: Interdisciplinary Team Development", McLean, VA: National Hospice Organization.

Vachon, M. L. S., Lyall, W. A. L., Rogers, J., Cochrane, J., and Freeman, S. J. J., 1981-1982, The effectiveness of psychosocial support during post-surgical treatment of breast cancer, International Journal of Psychiatry in Medicine, 11(4):365-372.

Vachon, M. L. S., Rogers, J., Lyall, W. A. L., Lancee, W. J., Sheldon, A. R., and Freeman, S. J. J., 1982, Predictors and correlates of high distress in adaption to conjugal bereavement, The American Journal of Psychiatry, 139(8):998-1002.

Weisman, A. D., 1981, Understanding the cancer patient: The syndrome of the caregiver's plight, Psychiatry, May 44:166-168.

White, W. L., 1978, "Incest in the Organizational Family: The Unspoken Issue in Staff and Program Burn-out", MD:HCI, Rockville.

Yancik, R., 1984, Sources of work stress for hospice staff, Journal of Psychosocial Oncology, 2(1):21-31.

Yancik, R., 1984, Coping with hospice work stress, Journal of Psychosocial Oncology, 22:19-35.

TERMINAL CARE OF THE CHILD WITH CANCER:

AN ANALYSIS OF PARENT/CHILD ATTITUDES

G.B. Humphrey, W.A. Kamps, E. de Bruin, H. Bosma and A. Kingma

Division of Pediatric Oncology
University Hospital
Groningen, The Netherlands

INTRODUCTION

At the time of initial diagnosis, it is common practice for one or more members of a pediatric oncology team to schedule a formal conference with the parents (and generally the patient). During such a conference the diagnosis, prognosis and treatment are discussed. The goal of initial therapy is to cure the child and thus at most pediatric oncology centers the child is generally treated according to a phase III research protocol.

Presently not all children with cancer will be cured. Unfortunately, at that time, it is not common practice for members of the team to discuss the imminence of death nor is there a commonly accepted definition of when terminal care begins.

During the initial conference explicit information is given, the process of informed consent is structured and the goals of therapy (the intent to maximise the possibility of curing the child with cancer) are clearly outlined. However, during the terminal phase the information given by physicians is not always as explicit as the information given at the time of diagnosis.

We have been interested in problems that relate to terminal care. One of the first questions is how to define the beginning of the terminal care phase. For the purpose of this study, we have defined this as the point in time when the oncology team decides that the child's cancer is no longer responsive (progressive disease or a relapse) to potentially curable (phase III) therapy. Then the child is eligible for treatment according to a phase II or phase I research protocol. As is well known to most individuals involved in terminal care, the goal of a phase II protocol is to determine which tumours will respond to new chemotherapeutic agents or new combinations of agents and the goal of a phase I protocol is to determine dose limiting toxicity of new agents. We have used this definition of terminal care in one prospective study of children and therapeutics (Nitschke et al, 1982) and two companion retrospective studies (Kamps et al., 1987; Humphrey, in press).

This paper will discuss and compare the attitudes of parents of children and children cured of cancer with regard to three issues:

1) whether the child should attend a terminal care conference,

2) whether the child should be involved in decisions and

3) whether the child alone should be allowed to give consent.

     While the parental part of this Dutch data base has already been pub-
lished (Kamps, et al., 1987) the age distribution data (from both parents and
children) has not been previously presented.

METHODS

     Parental attitudes were assessed by means of a mailed questionnaire as
previously reported (Kamps 1987). Briefly a questionnaire composed of 24
questions was sent to 156 Dutch parents, residents of the four northern
provinces of the Netherlands. Most parents considered it acceptable for
cured children to participate in a similar study, but only 25 children actually participated. This second study was conducted in the home as semi-
structured interview which included all components of the mailed parental
questionnaire. With regard to this study, parents and children were asked
questions about three areas of terminal care: as previously mentioned
should the child (1) attend a terminal care conference; (2) be involved in
decisions; (3) decide alone. Those individuals answering in the affirmative
were then asked at what age the child should be involved in these areas.
These two retrospective studies contain other information which has been used
to analyse issues in ethics, informed consent, experimental therapy, etc.
(Kamps et al., 1987; Humphrey, in press). The figures are presented as a
percentage of participants. Five childhood/adolescent age groups in years
were used for analysis and defined as follows: (1) 0-8, (2) 9-10, (3) 11-12,
(4) 13-14, (5) 15-19. Confidentiality was assured to both parents and child,
thus individual responses cannot be compared (i.e. parent-child disagreement
or agreement).

RESULTS

     Should the child attend a terminal phase conference?

     The responses to this question is given in figure 1. For those answer-
ing in the affirmative (see methods) the median age (range) at which the
child should attend was 12.1 yrs (4-19) parent preference and 10.5 yrs (3-15)
child preference. The distribution by age group is given in figure 2.

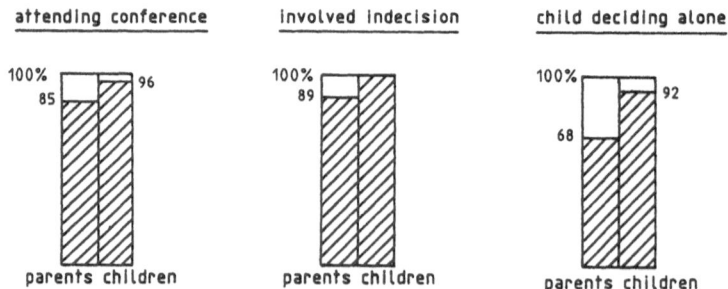

Figure 1. Parent child attitudes as to whether the child with recurrent
           resistant cancer should attend a terminal phase conference.
           Parent child attitudes towards: be involved in decisions.
           Parent child attitudes as to whether: give consent alone.

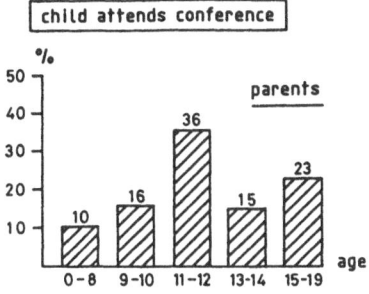

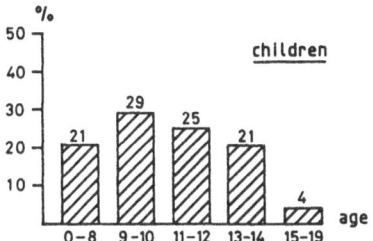

Figure 2.   Bar graph distribution of age groups in years for parents and
             for the child's opinion as to how old the child should be in
             order to attend the conference.

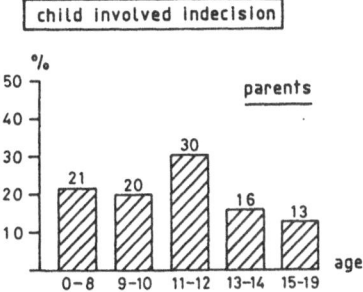

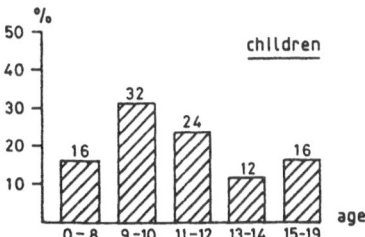

Figure 3.   Bar graph distribution of age groups in years for parents and
             for the child as to how old the child should be in order to be
             involved in decisions.

163

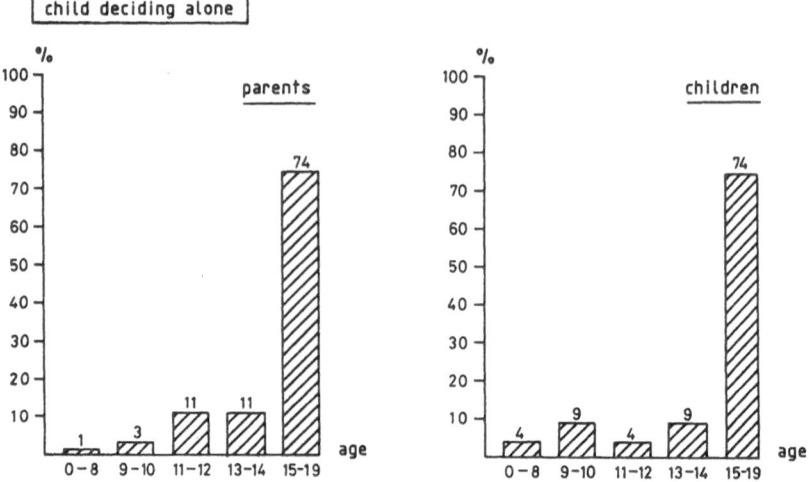

Figure 4.   Bar graph distribution of age groups in years for parents and
             for the child in order to give consent alone.

Should the child be involved in decisions?

    The response is given in figure 1. The parent/child preference as to
median (range) age for involvement was 11.8 years (4-19) and 11.6 years
(6-16) respectively. The distribution by age group is given in figure 3.

    Should the child alone decide the nature of terminal care?

    The response is given in figure 1 and the parent/child preferences were
15.8 years (7-19) and 15.5 years (8-19) respectively. The distribution by
age group is given in figure 4.

DISCUSSION

    The management of the terminal pediatric cancer patient remains a
significant problem. While approximately one half of children with cancer
can be cured, the other half will have progress in disease and require terminal care. While much has been written about terminal care of the child
with cancer, most of these reports are global reflections of extensive
personal experience with a few illustrative cases or they are case reports
from which global conclusions are drawn (Van Dongen 1986). Thus very few
structured studies exist in this field. Retrospective studies such as this
report give some insight into these problems but what is needed are random-
ized prospective studies in which data acquisition and/or intervention
strategies are conducted by one team and evaluation is done independently
by a second one.

    From our retrospective studies, it would appear that the majority of
both parents and children agree that the child should be involved to some
extent in terminal care decisions (fig. 1.) A simple comparison of the
median age at which the child should be involved in terminal care again
suggests agreement between parents and children. However, the age distribution data of involvement in a terminal care conference and involvement in
decision indicate that some parents would exclude children in the age range
9-14 years when in fact some children felt that children in this age range
should be included (fig. 2 and 3). This is of course not surprising.

Also there are two interesting observations with regard to the third area: the child decides alone. Again a greater percentage of children than parents thought the child alone should decide (fig. 1). However, the majority of respondents in the affirmative from both groups agreed that the adolescent (15 to 19 years) should decide alone on the nature of terminal care. This is in keeping with Dutch legal systems in that adolescents can obtain birth control prescriptions without parental consent, can obtain federal support for independent living arrangements, etc.

While statistics can be applied to these type of studies, this was not done in this analysis. The rationale for this decision was based on the large number of parents (137) and the relatively small number of children (25) interviewed. Whatever the limits of these studies are, we do feel strongly that they suggest or even require that we continue this area of inquiry. The insight given from these studies may be in part unique to the Dutch, but they are indeed intended for use in developing a prospective study of terminal care of Dutch children with cancer. Future advances in therapeutic research could of course eventually minimize the need for better terminal care.

REFERENCES

Humphrey, G. B., Kamps, W. A., Kingma, A., and Nitschke, R., Serial studies of informed consent in children, Biomedicine, in press.
Kamps, W. A., Akkerboom, J. C., Kingma, A., and Humphrey, G. B., 1987, Experimental chemotherapy in children with cancer - a parent's view, Pediatric Hematology and Oncology 4:117-124.
Nitschke, R., Humphrey, G. B., Sexauer, C. L. Catron, B., Wunder, S., and Jay, S., 1982, Therapeutic choices made by patients with end-stage cancer, J. Pediatr., 101:471-476.
Van Dongen, J. E. W. M., and Sanders-Woudstra, J. A. R., 1986, Psychosocial aspects of childhood cancer: a review of the literature, J Child Psychology and Psychiatry 27:145-80.

EVALUATION OF THE USE OF TERMINAL CARE SERVICES IN AN INNER CITY DISTRICT

C.M. McKee and G. Rajartnam

Department of Community Health
London School of Hygiene and Tropical Medicine
London, U.K.

INTRODUCTION

An inner London district health authority established a terminal care support service in 1983. The team comprised a hospital based team with two nursing sisters and informal support from three clinicians, and a community element consisting of a nursing sister in a co-ordinating role with district nurses.

The health authority has a resident population of approximately 150,000 and contains two acute hospitals with a total of 720 beds. Both hospitals are situated at the northern edge of the district and there is a large cross-boundary flow of patients between adjacent districts. The team had perceived that a number of patients who would benefit from their services were not being referred to them and many of those referred were seen at a late stage in their illness. The large cross boundary flow made it difficult to determine the potential number of patients who would be expected to come into contact with health services in the district. A study was therefore undertaken to examine what proportion of potential patients were being referred to the team. A further study examined the characteristics of those patients that were referred.

METHODS

Calculation of the proportion of potential patients referred was confined to those that were resident in the district. This was because these individuals could be easily identified from extracts of death certificates held within the district. As hospital activity analysis (HAA) data and team records had shown that district residents were slightly more likely to be referred than those living in other districts, the calculated figure would, if anything, tend to be an overestimation.

All death certificates of district residents dying over a six month period were examined. Details were extracted from all in which a malignant neoplasm (ICD-9 140-209) was mentioned.

These were cross referenced with the records of patients seen by the hospital and community teams during this period and the year preceding it.

RESULTS

229 district residents were found to have died from malignant disease, and 58 occurred in hospitals within the district. A further 40 took place at home. It was assumed that all patients dying at home would have had some contact with a hospital at some stage of their illness, and HAA data suggested that about 40% of these contacts would have been within the district. The number that might therefore have been referred to the team was calculated to be 74.

Of the total dying in district hospitals or at home, 26 (35%) had been referred.

14 (35%) of the 40 patients dying at home had been seen by the community team.

Comprehensive details about demographic characteristics were only available for those patients seen by the hospital team. Patients referred to the hospital team were slightly younger than those not seen (68 and 72 years respectively, p<0.05). Males and females were equally likely to be referred and the age distribution of those referred was similar. 55% of patients seen lived alone.

Comparison of referrals with the pattern of admissions of patients with malignant disease suggested that physicians were less likely to refer patients than were surgeons or gynaecologists. The pattern of sites of tumour among those referred was similar to that of all deaths in the district. Residents of the district constituted a higher proportion of referrals to the team than expected in relation to their representation among all admissions of patients with cancer to district hospitals, although there was no conscious policy to exclude patients from elsewhere.

Median survival following referral was 45 days and 25% of patients were referred in the week prior to death. Factors associated with late referral included being male, living alone, and old age.

The proportion of patients seen by the team who died at home was the same as among all patients dying of cancer in the district. Following referral the mean number of days spent in hospital was 30 days, and this was the same for patients living with relatives and those living alone. 25% of patients referred were admitted on more than one occasion and 4 were admitted more than 5 times.

DISCUSSION

This study provided information about the operation of the service and the factors associated with referral. A separate study had demonstrated a low level of awareness of the service and a lack of training in terminal care among other health workers in association with a perceived need for more assistance with terminal patients. This suggests that 35% is a sub-optimal level of referral.

Estimation of the proportion of patients dying from cancer who will be expected to require specialised care is difficult, although this information is important to anyone planning a service. We are only aware of one other similar study (Evans and McCarthy, 1984). It was carried out in a neighbouring district and it found that 55% of potential patients were seen. It did not use record linkage.

The scope of a service will depend upon pre-existing interest and expertise among health workers as well as socio-demographic factors such as the proportion of patients living alone.

The study emphasizes the requirement, in cities at least, to consider the effect of cross boundary patient flow when predicting need and assessing uptake of services. In this case if the number of cancer deaths occurring among district residents had been used as a denominator the result would have been misleading.

It also indicates a requirement for effective liaison with hospital and community services in neighbouring districts.

A substantial number of patients were referred at a very late stage in their illness. There are a number of reasons that might explain this, and some patients will inevitably die unexpectedly. The team had felt that in many cases they were only seeing patients when other health workers had given up and this did not give them enough time to stabilize the patient on effective treatment. Those patients that are referred earlier may have several stays in hospital over a period of time and it is essential that communication between clinicians and terminal care providers is good.

There is a considerable body of literature concerning the quality and management of terminal care services. We feel that there is a requirement for further epidemiological studies to assist with planning and evaluating services.

REFERENCES

Evans, C., and McCarthy, M., 1984, Referral and survival of patients accepted by a terminal care support team, J Epid Comm Health, 38:310-314.

THE EFFECTIVENESS OF A PSYCHOLOGICAL TRAINING DESIGNED FOR HEALTH CARE

PROFESSIONALS DEALING WITH TERMINAL CANCER PATIENTS

Nicole Delvaux, Darius Razavi, Christine Farvacques
and Edmond Robaye

Universite Libre de Bruxelles
Bruxelles, Belgium

INTRODUCTION

The medical and nursing staff can, through their listening attitude and their interventions, contribute to the psychosocial adaptions of the patient, as well as to maintaining the quality of life, in the terminal stage. In cancer care, as well as in terminal care, stressors are numerous. These stressors are summarized in Table 1.

However, general professional training remains essentially centred upon technical aspects without investigating the problems raised by the psychological issues of terminal cancer care. Psychological aid to the patient in the terminal stage, as well as to his family, rests with all staff in attendance, and is not limited to mental health professionals. Psychiatrists and psychologists have their part to play in making health care teams sensitive to these aspects of their work, and in their psychological education, (Stedford and Bloch, 1979).

Table 1.

USUAL STRESSORS IN TERMINAL CARE

---

* Numerous critical decisions even with ambiguous informations

* Highly consequent errors

* Numerous emotional contacts with patients/families

* Communication of bad news

* Numerous therapeutic failures/death

* Administration of aversive treatment with side effects

* Numerous contacts with mutilated/defigured patients

Table 2.   FACTORS WHICH COULD EXPLAIN THE EFFECTIVENESS OF PSYCHOLOGICAL
           TRAINING

---

* a better perception and recognition of patient and family needs

* the knowledge of interventions strategies

* the development of creativity and interest in research

* a positive attitude towards work, care and patients

* a sense of control on stress factors

* a transformation of the stress of caring in a satisfaction of care

* the development of a support network system

The importance of psychological training is often recognised, and rarely
put into practice. Elaboration of its content and form (nature, program
length, techniques and aims) varies with the experience and personal options
of the trainer. Interventions can be educational, and/or psychodynamic
(Bloom, 1975; Levington and Frets, 1978-79; Barton and Crowder, 1975;
Anderson, 1982; Kalish, 1985; Moore, 1984; Shanfield, 1981; Shinn et al.,
1984; Ziegler et al.,1984; Bertman et al., 1982; Campbell, 1980; Barstow,
1980). Training effectiveness can be evaluated by cognitive, emotional,
behavioral or attitudinal measures of change (Amaral et al., 1981; Miles,
1980; Craytor and Fass, 1982; Mullins and Merriam, 1983; Murray, 1974;
McClam, 1980; Gray-Toft, 1980; Liberman et al., 1983-84; Brown, 1981, Bensing
and Sluijs, 1984). Not enough has been done to evaluate the effectiveness
of such training. The susceptible factors which could explain this effectiveness are summarized in Table 2.

In a study evaluating a supportive, emotional and psychodynamic group
for oncology nurses, P.M. Silberfarb and P.M. Levine (1980) administered a
semantic differential scale to the group members and a comparison group,
before and after the sessions. They noted no significant differences
between the groups : the oncology nurses who had completed the group experience had meanwhile more negative attitude shifts to the job-pertinent
concepts and also showed a greater amount of attitude change in the negative
direction than those oncology nurses not in the group. On the basis of these
differences, the authors discussed the importance of denial in the daily
functioning of professionals working in cancer centers. Taking these findings into account, they suggested a pedagogical model to replace any emotional group process.

A first study was designed in order to evaluate the proposed pedagogical
model. A brief training approach was chosen in order to be as practical and
cost effective as possible. A second study was designed in order to have a
better understanding of the training process. This study includes for this
purpose a two month pre-training and a two month post-training assessment.

FIRST STUDY

1. METHODOLOGY

This study reports the evaluation of eighteen training groups for health
care professionals working in different institutions spread over the French
speaking part of Belgium. Most of them are general acute hospitals with

internal medicine and surgery departments or institutions for long term care. Four institutions provide home care.

The groups

All the participating subjects were self referred, or invited to participate by the institution's manager after an informative meeting. An informative meeting had been organized in each establishment setting out the objectives of the proposed training.

Motivations to attend the training groups were expressed by participants in terms of difficulty when facing the fatally ill and his family. Their expectations were to learn about what to tell to the patient and what kind of reactions are expected in these situations.

Different types of health care professionals participated to the training: nursing assistants, nurses, social workers, physicians, psychologists, physical therapists and also non professional volunteers and clergymen. A majority of the participants were nurses.

In all cases, the training was 12 hours in duration spread over 4, 6, 8 or 10 sessions. Each session lasted from 75 to 180 minutes : flexibility was required for the time available for training in each institution. The frequency of sessions varied with work schedules and holidays so that the sessions were sometimes spread over three months.

Each group was trained by the same person. For most it was a graduate psychologist, except for one group trained by a psychiatrist and six groups trained by two graduate psychologists working together.

Aims, content and techniques were similar across groups. The aims of the training was to develop a better understanding of the psychosocial aspects of terminal cancer care and to help these professionals to develop positive attitudes in their work. Training included role playing, comparing experiences, discussing cases and theoretical concepts. The first session was devoted to explaining the aims, techniques, and program of training, permitting participants to express their motivations for training. The content of the next meetings were case discussions, theoretical information and exchange about the terminal patient psychology, the family reactions and the health care professionals attitudes. Finally, information was given about terminal care in Belgium. The last meeting was devoted to an evaluation of the training by the participants and to setting their future expectations. Figure 1 summarized the repartition of cognitive, experiential, emotional and behavioral content of the training.

The subjects

The number of subjects who completed the training and the questionnaire was 122 (22 subjects did not complete the questionnaire : some of them refused, others did not complete the training). A comparison or control group of 43 subjects who came from five of these institutions completed the questionnaire but did not receive training.

Evaluation

The present study incorporates the semantic differential questionnaire designed by P.M. Silberfarb and P.M. Levine (1980) on the psychosocial aspects of cancer and applied in the context of supportive groups designed for oncology nurses. The contrasting adjectives of the semantic differential questionnaire remained constant for each concept scored and were chosen from the evaluative adjective scales compiled by Osgood, Suci, and Tannenbaum

(1971). The questionnaire was translated into French and adapted for the psychosocial aspects of fatal illness.

The questionnaire was given to the participants during the first and the last meetings of the training. In the comparison group, the second questionnaire was submitted two months following completion of the first questionnaire. The questionnaire consists of a list of 20 attitudes (Table 3), each of which must be located on 13 semantic differential scales. The 20 attitudes were grouped in five categories or concepts (Table 3).

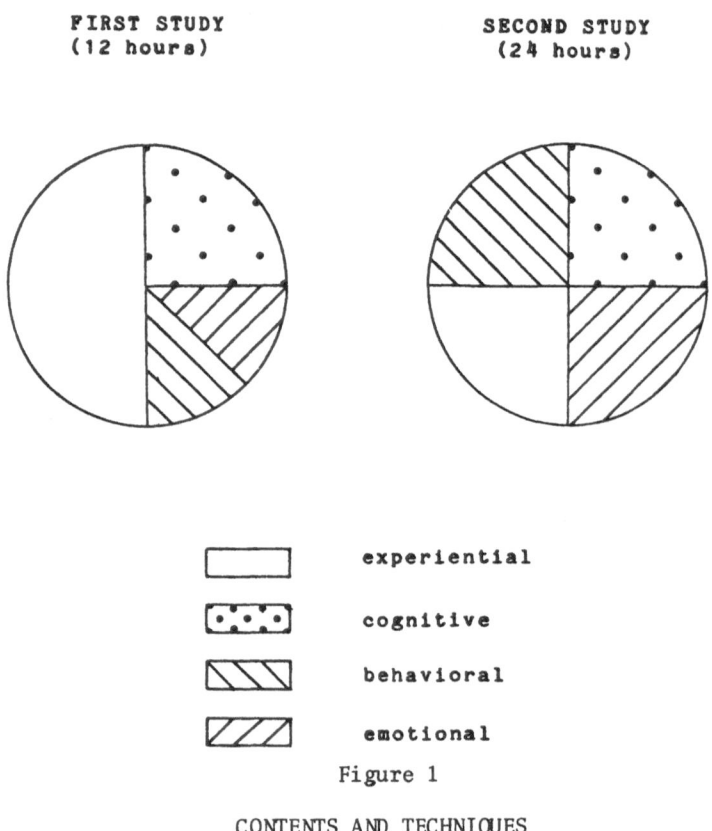

FIRST STUDY
(12 hours)

SECOND STUDY
(24 hours)

experiential

cognitive

behavioral

emotional

Figure 1

CONTENTS AND TECHNIQUES

USED IN THE TRAINING PROGRAM

The semantic differential scales are scored from 1 to 7 from the positive to the negative pole. By adding up the scores obtained from each question on the 13 scales, and then dividing them by 13, a score is obtained for each question. Score 4, 'neutral', is allotted whenever an answer is missing. For each subject, the scores attributed to the 20 attitudes are calculated to obtain a mean before training and a mean after training.

Table 3.

ATTITUDES AND CONCEPTS INVESTIGATED

Attitudes investigated

A1	Providing care for dying patient
A2	Quality of care
A3	Emotional growth as a result of working experience
A4	Professional relationship with the physicians
A5	Attitude toward myself as a health care professional
A6	Professional role with dying patient
A7	Providing care for young dying patient
A8	Professional relationship with staff
A9	Attitude toward illness
A10	Attitude toward myself
A11	Attitude toward death
A12	Providing care for a dying patient of the same age
A13	Professional relationship with the psychiatric team
A14	Providing care for seriously ill patients
A15	Personal relationship with the staff
A16	Providing care for a middle age dying patient
A17	Personal growth as a result of working experience
A18	Attitude toward fatal illness
A19	Providing care for the elderly dying patients
A20	Educational growth as a result of working experience

Concepts investigated

C1	Attitude about oneself (attitudes 2, 5, 6, 10)
C2	Attitude toward illness and death (attitudes 9, 11, 18)
C3	Personal growth (attitudes 3, 17, 20)
C4	Professional relationships (attitudes 4, 8, 13, 15)
C5	Occupational attitudes (attitudes 1, 7, 12, 14, 16, 19)

The validity of the questionnaire was tested on a sample of 199 subjects particularly for internal consistency and relevance. Item–total correlations were computed and these ranged from 0.303 to 0.805. Attitude related to professional relationship with the psychiatric team has the weakest correlations (0.303) because a majority of subjects didn't have this kind of professional relationship. All the correlations are highly significant ($p < 0.001$). To assess the factor structure of the semantic differential questionnaire, the data (199 questionnaires) were factor analyzed by Hotteling and Thurstone methods, (Faverge, 1954). Factor analysis by attitudes shows five factors corresponding, with at least two attitudes, to the five concepts. The five factors emerged accounting respectively for 67%, 17.9%, 5.6%, 5.2% and 4% of the variance. Factorial analysis realized for each concept shows one factor including all the questions related to the concepts. These results confirm the internal consistency of the semantic differential questionnaire and the relevance of the concepts.

Statistical analysis

Chi square test was used in order to compare control and training subjects for age, sex, marital status, experience and professional status.

A statistical analysis was carried out in order to test the attitude changes after training and the predictive value of positive and negative attitudes on the post training change (Dagnelie, 1975; D'Hainaut, 1975). This analysis was performed in the Brussels Free University Computer Center with the SPSS (Statistical Package for Social Sciences).

For each group (training and comparison) of subjects, a set of 20 indices was obtained, corresponding to attitude changes for the 20 questions. For each group of subjects, the 20 indices were grouped in five categories, which reflect attitudes about oneself (attitudes 2,5,6,10), toward fatal illness and death (attitudes 9,11,18), personal growth (attitudes 3,17,20), professional relationship (attitudes 4,8,13,15), and occupational attitudes (attitudes 1,7,12,14,19). For each of these five categories or concepts, an average index was obtained by averaging the indices of attitude changes for that category constituent attitudes.

The amount of attitude change after training was measured by the following formula : $di = d1 - d2$ ($d1$ = score before training, $d2$ = score after training). A negative di ($d1 < d2$) means a negative attitude change, as the highest values on the differential semantic scale of the questionnaire represents a negative attitude change.

For each attitude and concept, we carried out a dependent two-tailed t-test for each group (training and no training) of subjects, to test the level of significance of the difference observed when comparing the mean scores before and after the training.

Changes (training and comparison group) in attitudes were tested with an analysis of covariance (ANCOVA).

In order to analyse whether or not attitude (negative versus positive) at the beginning of the training could predict the attitude change after the training, a correlation analysis was performed between attitude global score before training and change due to training for the training and control group.

Further, subjects were divided in order to obtain a subgroup with negative attitudes and one with positive attitudes. The cut-off point chosen here was 3.04 (median of the whole sample). Subjects with negative attitudes had thus a mean global score before training higher than 3.04 and those with a positive attitude, a mean global score lower than 3.04. An analysis of covariance, and a two-tailed t-test for post training differences of these positive and negative subgroups was also performed.

2. RESULTS

There were no significant differences (chi square test) between control (n = 43) and trained subjects (n = 122) when compared for age, sex, marital status, education, professional status and experience with terminal patients.

The covariance analysis (ANCOVA) shows significant attitude change between training and control groups for the attitude four (A4) ($p = 0.022$) (Table 4).

The total attitudes scores moved significantly to the positive pole for the trained subjects only ($p < 0.01$). For this group, before and after, differences were significant (two-tailed dependent t-test) for eleven on a total of twenty items ($p < 0.01$; $p < 0.05$). For the control group, only three before-after differences were significant ($p < 0.05$); one attitude moved significantly to the negative pole ($p < 0.05$).

Table 4.   TRAINING GROUP EFFECTIVENESS FOR HEALTH CARE PROFESSIONALS

	before after differences (di)		tg / cg Comparison
	training group (tg) (N =122)	control group (cg) (N=43)	ANCOVA p value
A1	0.113	−0.157	0.069
A2	0.359 **	−0.011	0.949
A3	0.207 *	0.112	0.716
A4	0.227 *	0.010	0.022
A5	0.193	0.104	0.932
A6	0.231 **	−0.185	0.159
A7	0.258 *	0.220	0.906
A8	−0.011	−0.222	0.469
A9	0.173	0.025	0.439
A10	0.134	0.022	0.837
A11	0.285 **	0.298 *	0.680
A12	0.127	0.131	0.986
A13	0.079	0.156	0.851
A14	0.045	0.019	0.503
A15	0.230 **	−0.204	0.172
A16	0.072	0.023	0.996
A17	−0.040	−0.201 *	0.414
A18	0.218 **	0.057	0.827
A19	0.198 *	0.297	0.386
A20	0.167 *	0.130	0.727
C1	0.229 **	−0.017	0.317
C2	0.225 **	0.126	0.904
C3	0.111	0.014	0.479
C4	0.131 *	−0.065	0.074
C5	0.136 *	0.088	0.895
Total	0.163 **	0.031	0.366

* $p < 0.05$ (two-tailed) Student dependent t-test
** $p < 0.01$ (two-tailed) Student dependent t-test

The before-after differences for the trained subjects were significant for concepts one and two ($p < 0.01$), four and five ($p < 0.05$), and no before-after differences were significant for the controls subjects.

A significant relation was found between the pre-training attitude (defined as the global attitude between training for each health professional) and change due to training : Spearman correlation between attitudes before and before-after differences was significant ($r=0.41$; $p < 0.001$) for the training group and not significant ($r=0.16$) for the control group.

When comparing training and control groups with pre-training negative attitudes (Table 5), the analysis of covariance shows significant improvement differences for total score ($p < 0.02$), concepts 1 ($p < 0.02$) and 4 ($p < 0.001$), and six attitudes : A1, A4 ($p < 0.01$); A6, A10, A15, A20 ($p < 0.05$).

The before-after differences attitude changes (two-tailed dependent t-test) for the trained subjects in this negative attitudes subgroup were all positive and significant for thirteen on a total of twenty items : ten were significant at a 0.01 level and three at a 0.05 level. Concepts differences were all significant at a 0.01 level. All the post-training attitudes move to the positive pole ($p < 0.01$).

For the control subjects in the negative attitudes subgroup, the before-after attitude changes (two-tailed dependent t-test) were significant for attitudes 1, 8 and concept 4 at a 0.05 level.

When comparing training and control groups with pre-training positive attitudes, the analysis of covariance shows a significant change only for attitude 19 ($p < 0.02$).

In the training subgroup with pretraining positive attitudes, no before-after attitude changes (two-tailed dependent t-test) were significant but twelve on a total of twenty items were more negative. In the control sub-group with pre-training positive attitudes, attitude changes were significantly positive for A11 and A19 ($p < 0.05$) and significantly negative for A17 ($p < 0.01$). Table 5 summarizes these results.

Globally, the participants and leader subjective evaluation about the training concurs with the statistical results. The participants expressed their satisfaction at the end of the training : it had helped them to a better understanding of the situation; a majority felt rather more reassured about the subject itself, even if they were still apprehensive about the situation. All of the participants felt that the training was too short. In three training groups, a continuation of the training was proposed.

3. DISCUSSION

When the subjects are considered globally, the attitude changes are limited to a positive improvement of professional relationship with physicians. This trend is confirmed by the move of the concept four. It is interesting to underline that for an emotional training group the same attitude was moving negatively (Silberfarb and Levine, 1980). Attitudes about oneself are also moving positively showing a non specific effect of the training. These limited and non specific training effects could be explained by the short duration of the training assessed here or by problems related to the tool used here for the assessment of the effectiveness. They are however, when considered together with the subjective assessment of the trainers and the trained, important to be emphasized.

The positive attitude change found here shows the relevance of the pedagogical training program. The effectiveness of a pedagogical approach does not necessary mean that there was no emotional reactions involved in the group process and that this should be avoided in order to improve effectiveness. Improving effectiveness may also be achieved by a longer training process. Longer training will probably have a deeper impact on the participants.

This study shows a remarkable effectiveness of short training groups for health care professionals dealing negatively (with negative attitudes) with terminal patients. The different training effect for subjects with negative attitudes when compared to those with positive attitudes are challenging for the theorization about the potential benefits and risks.

There is a need to have a better understanding about factors which could predict a significant change. This will allow to design special training for 'resistant' subjects with regard to their style or personality. The fact that those who have negative attitudes were good subjects is a first step for that purpose but the meaning of positive and negative attitudes need to be investigated. Are those who report good attitudes deniers or subjects who have already developed (successfully?) coping mechanisms in order to deal with dying patients? In this study the change is meaningful but does it also assess behavior modifications when dealing with patients.

Table 5.   NEGATIVE ATTITUDE : A PREDICTOR OF TRAINING EFFECTIVENESS

	Subjects with positive attitudes			Subjects with negative attitudes		
	before after differences		tg / cg comparison	before after differences		tg / cg comparison
	training group (tg) (N=53)	control group (cg) (N=27)	ANCOVA p value	training group (tg) (N=69)	control group (cg) (N=16)	ANCOVA p value
A1	-0.004	-0.070	0.461	0.202 **	-0.304 *	0.008
A2	0.113	0.108	0.450	0.547 *	-0.211	0.412
A3	0.117	0.211	0.916	0.277 **	-0.054	0.232
A4	0.089	0.186	0.289	0.333 **	-0.287	0.001
A5	0.090	0.143	0.626	0.271 **	0.038	0.211
A6	-0.014	-0.101	0.785	0.420 **	-0.327	0.035
A7	0.167	0.299	0.747	0.329 *	-0.087	0.361
A8	-0.097	-0.083	0.720	0.056	-0.457 *	0.057
A9	0.154	-0.001	0.561	0.187	-0.068	0.944
A10	-0.021	0.118	0.142	0.252 **	-0.138	0.046
A11	0.136	0.382 *	0.472	0.400 **	0.155	0.276
A12	0.171	0.289	0.943	0.093	-0.133	0.279
A13	-0.026	0.155	0.682	0.160	0.158	0.630
A14	-0.179	-0.015	0.589	0.217	0.058	0.717
A15	-0.036	-0.070	0.733	0.435 **	-0.432	0.014
A16	-0.153	0.090	0.294	0.244 *	-0.091	0.115
A17	-0.183	-0.362 **	0.704	0.069	0.072	0.390
A18	-0.037	-0.128	0.841	0.414 **	0.368	0.751
A19	-0.125	0.460 *	0.017	0.447 **	0.022	0.060
A20	-0.041	0.084	0.377	0.326 **	0.208	0.032
C1	0.042	0.066	0.490	0.373 **	-0.159	0.012
C2	0.084	0.084	0.758	0.334 **	0.197	0.570
C3	-0.035	-0.023	0.863	0.246 **	0.075	0.143
C4	-0.018	0.047	0.953	0.255 **	-0.255 *	0.001
C5	-0.020	0.175	0.314	0.255 **	-0.060	0.056
Total	0.006	0.085	0.601	0.284 **	-0.060	0.013

* p < 0.05 (two-tailed Student dependent t-test
** p < 0.01 (two tailed) Student dependent t-test

It is interesting enough also to note the positive trend observed over a two or three month period for subjects with positive attitudes who did not participate in a training group, and a negative trend for those with negative attitudes. This negative attitude change may be a correlation of the development of burnout already described for health care professionals (Maslach and Jackson, 1982).

Other instruments seem necessary to assess changes consequent to the training of health care professionals. Actually, only a small number of validated instruments measuring the effectiveness of training are available. Semantic differential questionnaires are one of these few's and is easy to use; our results show high internal consistency allowing further development and adaptations.

SECOND STUDY

A second study was designed in order to have a better understanding of the training process. The previous findings of an overall effectiveness made possible this longitudinal study aimed at assessing pre-training and post-training changes including the possible consolidation which may occur after the end of the program.

1. THE GROUPS, THE EVALUATION AND THE STATISTICAL ANALYSIS

Recruitment of subjects, of the second study is similar to the 15 health care professionals working in different institutions completed a four point assessment study : two months before training, at the first training session, at the last session and the two months after. The assessment includes the semantic differential questionnaire described here above.

The content and duration of the training program assessed in the second study was changed. The duration of the training remained short but was extended to 24 hours, spread over 8 weekly sessions. The content of the cognitive (didactic) program content didn't change. The behavioral and experiential content of the program were extended. The training has a cognitive (25%), behavioral (25%), emotional (25%) and experiential (25%) repartition. The cognitive work proposed to the participants is a didactic program (mainly theoretical informations). Behavioral training includes role playing sessions with a videotape and group feedback. The videotape and the group feedbacks include also experiential exchanges. The emotional work does not include an active emotional expression program. Emotional expressions are not stimulated, but the trainers do not inhibit the spontaneous emotional expressions when appearing during the course of the training.

The figure 1 shows the repartitions of techniques in the first and the second study. Attitudes and concept changes were statistically tested by a one tailed student t-test.

2. RESULTS

The results are showing some hypothesis we made and some unexpected ones: pre-training attitude changes as expected, were not significant. A pre-training positive change of the concept 2 (illness/death attitude) was however found. Even with a small sample, post-training changes reach the level of significance showing either an immediate post-training change ($p < 0.005$) and a consolidation two months later ($p < 0.025$).

Immediate training effectiveness was found for all the concepts. Two months post-training consolidation was not found for concept one (self concept) concept three (personal growth). Figure 2 shows the concept changes observed before and after training.

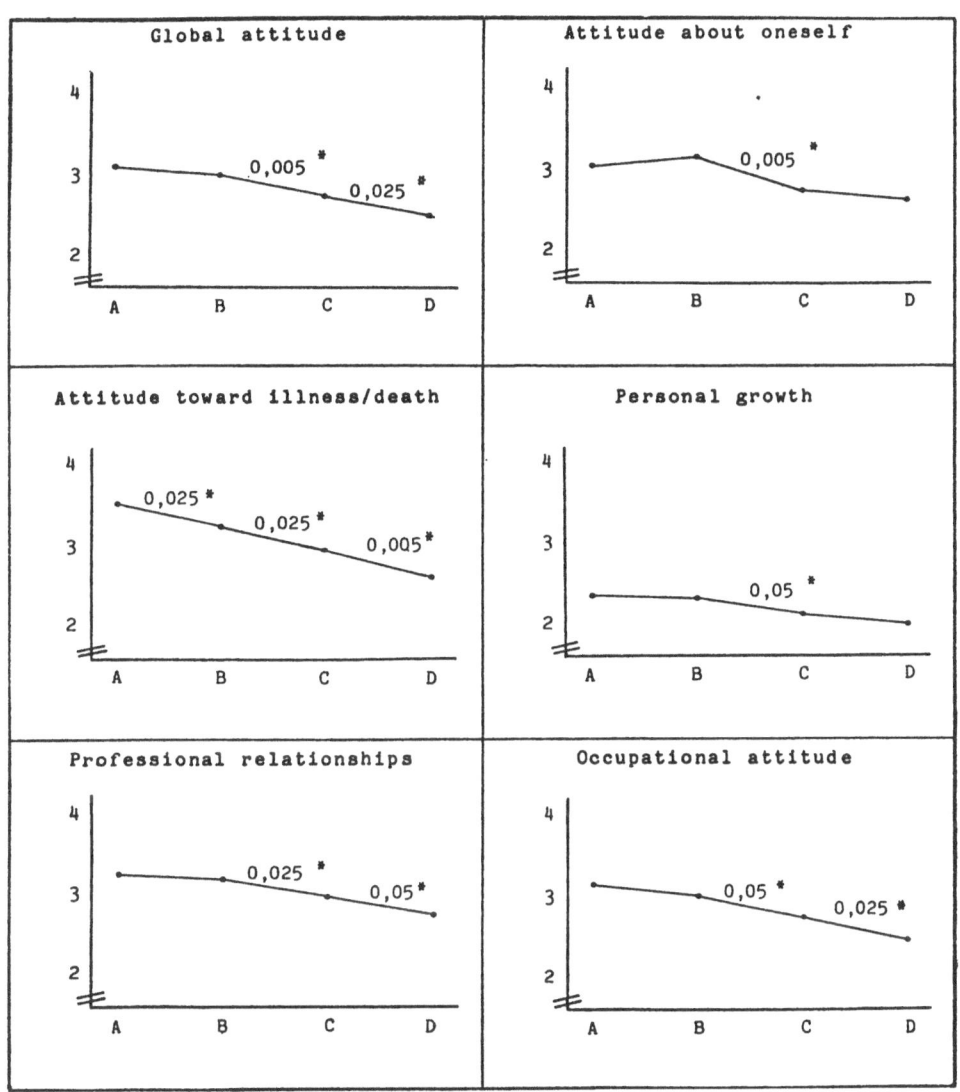

Figure 2

LONGITUDINAL ATTITUDES CHANGES
N = 15
(Mean Scores)

A : 2 months before training
B : first day training
C : last day training
D : 2 months after training

* p value (student t-test)

3. DISCUSSION

This second study confirms the first study showing the effectiveness of brief training groups for health care professionals dealing with terminal cancer patients. It gives some information about a possible post-training consolidation.

The training assessed in the second study, even longer (24 versus 12 hours), can be considered as brief, making them easy to be applied for students and for professionals working in institutions.

The absence of pre-training change is another way to prove, in a longi-tudinal design, the effectiveness of brief training programs. The interpre-tation of the pre-training significant change for concept 2 (attitudes towards illness and death) is difficult because of the small sample tested here and because of the need to increase and improve confidence in the psychometric properties of the semantic differential questionnaire.

We need also to be careful about a too quick interpretation of the absence of post-training consolidation for concept one (self concept) and concept three (personal growth).

CONCLUSION

Working with terminal cancer patients is a chronic stress and the health care professionals must be helped in order to develop coping strategies for maintaining quality of work and care. The principle of a psychological training in terminal care is beginning to be recognized as important but its content, forms and effectiveness needs further investigation.

Training groups, even brief, increase the possibility for health care professionals to get more information about issues related to death and dying and allow them to recognize similar attitudes in others.

Many questions are still raised with regard to the purpose of the training. Our program seems especially useful for health care professionals dealing negatively with dying patients. But meaning of this predictive factor has to be investigated.

This first controlled study shows the effectiveness of a short pedagogi-cal training program. Generalizing the use of such trainings in medical settings will probably improve the quality of care, and the quality of life of patients dealing with life threatening illness. The short duration of the training program make its use easy in various medical settings.

The problem of consolidation or long term effectiveness is an important question in the design of a training program for health care professionals. This question has particular significance when discussing the issue of the effectiveness of a brief training group.

The significant consolidation found here for a brief training group is one more argument to help health care professionals to cope with stressor met with in terminal care situations.

In the particular setting of terminal care, it allows better recognition of patients needs and gives the opportunity to use strategies in order to give appropriate response to them. Moreover, training, in our point of view, improves creativity in clinical work and interest in research issues. These benefits of training are reflected by a positive change in attitude about oneself, illness and death, personal growth and interpersonal professional relationship.

These are certainly not the only benefit of training. Other potential benefits are important to recall : the positive perception of work (care) and the creation of a network support system. These issues should also be assessed in future research.

A second generation of studies should aim at assessing effectiveness of training programs not only by change in attitudes but by quality of care as reflected in patients reported quality of life. The ultimate goal of a psychological training should of course be the satisfaction of patients with the care received.

ACKNOWLEDGEMENT

This research was supported by a grant of the 'Direction Generale de la Sante du Ministere de la Communaute Francaise' number 86/61836.

REFERENCES

Amaral, P., Nehemkis, A. M. and Fox, L., 1981, Staff support on a cancer ward: a pilot project, Death Education, 5:267-274.
Anderson, J. L., 1982, Evaluation of practical approach to teaching about communication with terminal cancer patients, Med. Educ., 16:202-207.
Barstow, J., 1980, Stress variance in hospice nursing, Nursing Outlook, December: 751-754.
Barton, D., and Crowder, M., 1975, The use of role playing techniques as an instructional aid in teaching about dying, death, and bereavement, Omega, 6:243-250.
Bensing, J., and Sluijs, E., 1984, Leren luisteren, maar wat dan? Evaluatie van een gesprekstraining voor huisartsen, Ned. Tijdschr. Psychol. 39:265-280.
Bertman, S. L., Greene, H. and Wyatt, C. A., 1982, Humanistic health care education in a hospice/palliative care setting, Death Education, 5:391-408.
Bloom, S., 1975, On teaching an undergraduate course on death and dying, Omega, 6:223-226.
Brown, I., 1981, The effects of a death education program for nurses working in a long-term hospital, Dissertation Abstracts International, 42:54.
Campbell, T. W., 1980, Death anxiety on a coronary heart unit, Psychosomatics, 21:127-136.
Craytor, J. K., and Fass, M. L., 1982, Changes nurses' perceptions of cancer and cancer care, Cancer Nursing, February:43-49.
Dagnelie, P., 1969, "Théorie et Methodes Statiques", Duculot, Gembloux.
D'Hainaut, L., 1975, "Concepts et Methodes de la Statistique", Labor, Bruxelles.
Faverge, J. M., 1954, "Méthodes Statistiques en Psychologie Appliquee", Tome Second, PUF, Paris.
Gray-Toft, P., 1980, Effectiveness of a counselling support program for hospice nurses, Journal of Counselling Psychology, 27:346-354.
Kalish, R. A., 1985, "Death, Grief and Caring Relationships", Second Edition, Brooks, Monterey.
Leviton, D. and Frets, B., 1978-79, Effects of education of fear of death and attitudes towards death and life, Omega, 9:267-277.
Liberman, M. B., Handal, P. J., Napoli, J. G. and Austrin, H. R., 1983-1984, Development of a behavior rating scale for doctor-patient interactions and its implications for the study of death anxiety, Omega, 14:231-239.
Maslach, C. H. and Jackson, S. E., 1982, Burnout in health professions: a social psychological analysis, in "Social Psychology of Health and Illness (Edited by G.S. Sanders and J. Suls), Laurence Erlbaum Associates, London.

McClam, T., 1980, Death anxiety before and after death education: negative
    results, Psychol. Rep., 46:513-514.
Miles, M. S., 1980, The effects of a course on death and grief on nurses'
    attitudes towards dying patients and death, Death Education, 4:245-260.
Moore, K., 1984, Training social workers to work with the terminally ill,
    Health and Social Work, 9:268-273.
Mullins, L. C. and Merriam, S., 1983, The effects of a short-term death
    training program on nursing home staff, Death Education, 7:353-368.
Murray, P., 1974, Death education and its effects on the death anxiety
    levels of nurses, Psychol. Rep., 35:1250.
Osgood, C. E., Suci, G. J. and Tannenbaum, P., 1971, "The Measurement of
    Meaning", University of Illinois Press, Chicago.
Shanfield, S. B., 1981, The mourning of health care professionals: an
    important element in education about death and loss, Death Education,
    4:385-395.
Shinn, M., Rosario, M., Morch, H., and Chestnut, D. E., 1984, Coping with
    job stress and burnout in human services, J. Pers. Soc. Psychol.,
    46:864-876.
Silberfarb, P. M., and Levine, P. M., 1980, Psychosocial aspects of
    neoplastic disease. III, Group support for the oncology nurse, Gen.
    Hosp. Psychiatr.,3:192-197.
Stedeford, A., and Bloch, S., 1979, The psychiatrist in the terminal care
    unit, Brit. J. Psychiat., 35:1-6.
Ziegler, J. L., Kanas, N., Strull, W. M., and Bennet, N., 1984, A stress
    discussion group for medical interns, J. Med. Educ., 59:205-207.

HEALTH SERVICES USED BY CANCER PATIENTS DURING THE TERMINAL THREE MONTHS

F.W. Gunz and I. Reynolds

Department of Clinical Oncology
Royal North Shore Hospital
St.Leonards, Australia

The Australian population has just passed the 16 million mark, and as Australians live in an expanse as large as the United States, you will guess that they may present problems in palliative care which differ in some ways from those in more densely settled parts of the world. However, for city dwellers the differences are smaller. The present study included no country patients. We worked in Sydney, which now has some 3.5 million people in its urban area, but there were rather fewer in 1982, the year on which our study was based, The reason why we had to go so far back was that our under-computerized Cancer Registry could give us no more recent figures. Our patients were investigated posthumously. They had all been seen at the Royal North Shore Hospital, which is an 800 bed teaching hospital with excellent oncology services, other than those for palliative care. Within its patient catchment area there were also two terminal care hospitals - I hesitate calling them hospices at that stage - with altogether 75 beds. The reason-ably well organised community services, including domiciliary nursing services, were then still getting into their full stride, and so their extent was not universally known. Altogether in 1982 palliative care was far less developed in Australia than in this country, but we have tried hard since then to catch up.

The investigation was planned as an attempt to test one of the common arguments that are used to justify demands for better domiciliary services: we are told that, because such services make longer home care possible, they not only give dying patients a better quality of life but also reduce the overall cost of caring for them. To us it seemed that, though there might be a cost benefit when one compared straight domiciliary with straight hospital care, this might be illusory because few patients were likely to be treated only at home or only in hospital during the terminal period. Probably there was some of each: they all started their medical career in hospital, but we knew little about the medical services they had used between that initial stage and their death. Putting it quantitatively, had patients who eventually died at home had less or more care, including hospital care, than their colleagues who spent their final days or weeks in an institution? That was the question we set out to answer.

Cancer is a notifiable disease in New South Wales, and particulars of our patients were obtained from the Cancer Registry. The sample consisted of all those patients who had died at home from cancer of the lung, colon or rectum during 1982 and who had been previously treated at the Royal

North Shore Hospital (Table 1). There were 34 of them, but because of imperfect records, we could only use 28. As controls we had 68 patients – two for each of the original names – who had died from the same cancers in institutions, also during 1982, and were also previously treated at Royal North Shore Hospital. They were matched with the sample for age, sex and diagnosis. I should add that overall, in New South Wales, only 12 - 15 % of cancer patients have died at home in recent years, and this was also true at our hospital.

More than half the control patients had died in the Royal North Shore Hospital (Table 2), the place where they were first treated, another quarter in the local terminal care hospitals and the rest in other hospitals or in nursing homes.

From the case notes we extracted details of all admissions during the three months preceding death. They ranged from none to five per patient, and the total of the days these patients spent in all institutions ranged from none to over 90. Table 3 shows numbers of days according to the place of death. It can be seen that half of the patients who died at home had not been admitted to any institution during the last three months of life. Only six of them (21%) spent more than 20 days in an institution, and none more than 50 days. But of those who died in institutions, over half had total admissions adding up to more than 20 days and 15% to more than 50 days. Clearly therefore patients who died at home had fewer institutional admissions during the pre-terminal period, and most of these were shorter than those of patients who died in institutions.

Table 1.   PATIENTS IN THE STUDY

DIAGNOSIS	DIED AT HOME	DIED IN INSTITUTION	TOTAL
CA LUNG	21	51	72
CA COLON	6	15	21
CA RECTUM	1	2	3
TOTAL	28	68	96

Table 2.   PLACE OF DEATH OF CONTROL PATIENTS

INSTITUTION	NUMBER	PERCENT
RNSH	37	54.4
OTHER GEN. HOSP.	4	5.9
TC HOSP.	16	23.5
PRIVATE HOSP.	9	13.2
NURSING HOME	2	2.9
TOTAL	68	99.9

Table 3.   INSTITUTIONAL DAYS IN TERMINAL THREE MONTHS

PLACE OF DEATH	DAYS ADMITTED					
	0	1-9	10-19	20-49	50-90+	TOTAL
HOME	14	4	4	6	0	28
RNSH	0	9	7	17	4	37
TC HOSP.	0	4	5	5	2	16
OTHER	0	4	2	5	4	15
TOTAL	14	21	18	33	10	96

What were the main reasons for these admissions? We were able to get them for the great majority (Table 4). Nearly half were for the relief of symptoms and fewer than a third for diagnosis or treatment. This made us think that better control of symptoms at home might have prevented the need for many of the admissions.

The next stage in our investigation was to find out what professional care, other than institutional, these people had had. To get an idea on this, we looked at hospital outpatients records and the notes of the community nurses, and we tried to contact every general practitioner who was listed in the case notes. This was much more difficult than extracting inpatient notes, and the information we got was less complete. In one third of cases, for instance, we could not determine if or how often, patients had seen their GP's, and in 1 to 8 cases there was uncertainty about the visits of home nurses. To our surprise nearly half had not been to the outpatients department in the terminal three months, 28% had not been in touch with their GP's, and as many as 80% had apparently failed to use our home nursing services. All these services were available but they were not used. As we did not interview the surviving relatives, we could not determine why the usage was so low. We suspect that in a good many cases, the reason was a lack of information on these services and how they could be obtained.

Table 4.   MAIN REASON FOR ADMISSIONS

REASON	ADMISSIONS	
	NUMBER	PERCENT.
SYMPTOM RELIEF	65	46.1
DIAGNOSIS	10	7.1
THERAPEUTIC	34	24.1
INTERCURRENT DISEASE	11	7.8
RESPITE, SOCIAL	18	12.8
OTHER	3	2.1
TOTAL	141	100.0

Table 5. TOTAL AVERAGE BED DAY COST PER PATIENT BY PLACE OF DEATH

PLACE OF DEATH	DAYS IN HOSPITAL	COST (£)
HOME	9.6	955
RNSH	24.5	2438
TC HOSP.	15.1	1506
1 DAY = £100		

We continue our investigations by firstly calculating inpatient costs using known bed-day costs at the various institutions. We also worked out what we called the direct in- and outpatient costs for each patient. They included consultations, anaesthetics, diagnostic and therapeutic procedures, pathology tests and intravenous therapy, all on the basis of the official Schedule of Health Services Benefits. The cost of drugs we calculated according to the figures in the Royal North Shore Hospital formulary. Costs of general practitioner and home nursing services were based on official unit fees. All these figures were expressed in terms of 1985 dollars, converted into pounds sterling.

In Australia, as no doubt in the United Kingdom, inpatient treatment is expensive. In our material, counting all the days which these patients spent in the various hospitals with their varying bed-day costs, the average daily cost per patient came to just about £100, the total for all admissions to £2,500 and the 'direct' costs to £600. The way this worked out for each of the groups is shown above (Table 5). You will see that the total cost for the 'home' group was about 40% and that for the 'terminal care hospital' group about 60% of that at the Royal North Shore Hospital. There was certainly no indication that patients who died at home had been unduly heavy hospital users previously. Nor did they make inordinate demands on out-patient or community services. Because our information on some of them was incomplete (Table 6), compared with inpatient costs, all others were rela-tively insignificant. They amounted between them to only 12.6% of all costs. These are of course averages. In some individual cases the cost of community services was much higher.

Table 6. TOTAL COSTS PER PATIENT (AVERAGE ALL PATIENTS USING SERVICE)

SERVICE	COST (£)	% OF TOTAL
INPATIENT	2555	87.4
OUTPATIENT	113	3.9
GP	82	2.8
HOME NURSING	174	5.9
TOTAL	2924	100.0

The three highest GP bills of up to £250 went to patients who died at home. Home nursing services cost up to £300 in individual cases but, perhaps because of the low usage, there was no clear overall relationship between place of death and cost. As a rough estimate, for those patients who died at home and who made maximal use of community services, the cost of these services might have amounted to about one half of the inpatient costs.

To sum up, the answer to the question we posed seems to be that our patients with terminal cancer who completed their days at home used fewer medical services and at a lower cost than those others who died in institutions. However, our study was something of a snapshot of a selected population at a particular time, and its wider relevance cannot be automatically assumed. We must especially ask what determined the places of death in our two main groups of patients who all came initially from the same hospital population, and whom we had been careful to match for other factors such as type of cancer, age, sex and date of death. Why did a few stay home to die when most did not? Were these in fact all members of a single population? If so, this must be very skewed in at least one respect, for we know that, overall, only 1 in 8 died at home. If indeed this was a single population, it could be argued that, by manipulations such as making home support services stronger and better known, more members might be induced to opt for the home, with consequent cost benefits. This change to home deaths, when support services were improved, has in fact occurred here and there including, I believe, parts of Scotland and even in Australia. However, the reversal has everywhere been only partial, and there is good evidence that, at least so far, the majority of deaths have continued to occur in hospitals and hospices. They may well do so in future, perhaps because there are in fact two populations who differ fundamentally according to where they choose, or are forced, to die. If true, it would supply a strong reason for continued pressure to improve all terminal care services, in- and outpatient, wherever they may be given.

PHYSICIAN'S ATTITUDES IN THE MANAGEMENT OF TERMINALLY ILL PATIENTS

G. Morasso, F. Cianfriglia, N. Crotti, F. De Falco
and M. Tamburrini

Istituto Tumori
Genova, Italy

INTRODUCTION

Communication between doctor and patient becomes particularly important where serious illnesses such as cancer are concerned, where conditioning and reactions are often less than rational.

In the opinion of a number of investigators, patients suffering from terminal illnesses should not be informed. This is based on the assumption that patients do not generally want to know that they are dying (Brim et al., 1970; Glaser and Strauss, 1965; Ley, 1977).

In other studies, such a decision ought to be determined on an individual level and based on factors such as I.Q., emotional state, social and cultural background, family backing and coping mechanism (Baanson, 1975; Hoerni and Lagarde, 1983; Reise, 1983).

Criteria determining when and how much the patient should know depends on the doctor/patient relationship. On the other hand, medical training provides rather scanty or non-existent guidelines for aiding patients in such circumstances (Holland, 1973; Novak, 1979; Reynolds et al., 1981).

In an earlier study carried out by us where 1st and 6th year medical students were compared, we were able to note how the attitude towards a cancer patient changed over the period of these years of study. The results of our study highlighted a progressive change in the image and role of the future doctor: 1st year students identified more with the patient and became emotionally involved in the relationship with him or her; students in their 6th year, on the other hand, tended to discard the image of medicine as a whole, favouring instead an overestimation of scientific possibilities and the necessity of a technical and instrumental knowledge together with a refusal of whatsoever personal involvement with the patient.

From these and other research (Poole and Sanson-Fisher, 1979; Reynolds et al., 1981), it becomes clear that there is an ever-growing importance, within doctor/patient communication, of factors which are not easily defin-able, such as the doctor's personality and consequently his own personal attitude to the clinical situation of the cancer patient. Other factors include a choice of the type of treatment, more or less aggressive, and the doctors ability to cope with his personal feelings of impotence in the face of death.

Doctors tend to take on a double role regarding cancer and death (Poole and Sanson-Fisher, 1979): both as men, with their fears and anxieties as regards death, and as doctors, professionally involved with their patients, with all the related responsibilities and decisions. Both of these human and professional levels do necessarily overlap and intertwine.

Within the professional doctor-cancer patient province, another variable to be considered is the different role and relevant expectations undertaken according to the different field of activity. This strongly conditions attitudes towards patients as research in the influence of professional experience and attitudes testifies (Blanchard, 1981; Hays, 1985; Krant, 1976; Ley, 1977).

PURPOSE

As stated in the introduction, the objective of the research consisted in analyzing the attitude of a sample of Italian physicians towards cancer patients in the terminal phase and in singling out to what degree such an attitude was conditioned by personal factors : sex and age; by sociocultural factors; or by the professional role.

METHODOLOGY

A 62-item multiple choice answer questionnaire was used. This was based on the Cancer Attitudes Questionnaire, completed by Haley and Blanchard in the U.S.A. (1981) and reproposed in France by Hoerni (1983).

We discussed the questionnaire with a group of 20 physicians, (oncologists, general practitioners, hospital practitioners, psychologists) in order to obtain the guidelines necessary for a more relevant re-elaboration which would better suit the Italian health system.

Some important points emerged from this discussion. Previous research studies used a 9 point answer evaluation scale (ranging from -4 in the case of absolute disagreement and +4 for complete agreement). From our discussion it emerged that the wider the possibility of choice, above all in highly emotive questions, the more doctors tended to answer briefly or give neutral responses ("I suppose I agree").

We therefore decided to devise a questionnaire based on statements allowing for only 3 possible responses: I AGREE (I believe this statement to be true), I DISAGREE (I believe this statement to be false) and I DON'T KNOW. Furthermore, we added some statements to the base questionnaire and left others out to make it more coherent with our research objectives and to make it more pertinent to the reality in our country. While carrying out this study, we also analysed the bibliography.

POPULATION

In collaboration with the 4 Cancer National Institutes (Milan, Rome, Naples and Genoa) we distributed 1,200 questionnaires to physicians in various cities in Italy, 655, equal to 54.5% were returned (The percentages of the results obtained are similar to those given in other studies). Using a random statistic criterion, we extracted a sample of 480 physicians (381 male, 99 female), in order to maintain an equal distribution in the 3 professional groups subdivided as follows:

                    160 family doctors
                    160 attending physicians (from various fields)
                    160 specialists in oncology

    The questionnaire was anonymous, self-completing, with a personal data
form and a letter of presentation and collaboration request. The aim of the
letter was to obtain greater involvement and enhance willingness to collabor-
ate. The questionnaires were distributed in 3 ways: 1) personal contacts
within the 4 National Cancer Institutes, 2) by post, using lists provided by
the various 'Ordini dei Medici' (Orders of Physicians), 3) during updating
courses for various professional categories. Compilation was individual and
without a deadline.

RESULTS

    The following study was carried out on the data collected: we grouped
the 62 statements under 5 attitudes we were interested in analysing.

(1) Attitude towards duty to inform or not on diagnosis, prognosis and
    therapy;
(2) Attitudes of physicians towards performing or not aggressive therapies
    on patients;
(3) Attitudes of physicians towards patients' resources face-to-face with
    cancer;
(4) Attitude towards death;
(5) Attitude towards the assumption or not of responsibilities to the patient
    and the dying person on the part of families, society and the physician.

    The responses given by those who completed the questionnaire were then
subdivided into 3 groups corresponding to the three professional categories
which were the object of the study:

                    - family doctors
                    - attending physicians (at the hospital)
                    - specialists - oncologists

    The choice percentages (%) were then calculated for each single state-
ment of:
                         - TRUE
                         - FALSE
                         - DON'T KNOW
                         - NONE

    Statistical processing was performed using X2 for each of the 5 attitudes
and for each single statement, comparing the 3 groups of physicians.

- we then calculated the mean of the answer percentages for each single
  attitude;
- then, an examination of the mean percentages of each group considered was
  performed;
- at this point a comparison between the various means of the 3 professional
  groups for each single attitude was carried out.

    A nominal scale of the 'certainty' (at non-regular intervals) with which
the physicians 'family doctors, attending physicians and oncologists) agreed
with our statements, was then constructed. The items were then ordered
(Rank Order) according to the choice percentages of 'true' responses where
'true' responses were greater than 50%. For greater visual clarity the
scales were reported in histograms.

Table 1. AGE DISTRIBUTION OF DOCTORS

Age	Family Doctors n.160 %	Attending Physicians n.160 %	Oncologists n.160 %	Total n.480 %
≤ 30	16.46	15.09	26.45	19.28
31–40	42.41	52.83	48.39	47.88
≥ 41	41.14	32.08	25.16	32.84

Table 2. PHYSICIAN/SEX RATIOS OF DOCTORS

Physicians	Males %	Females %
Family Doctors	86.25	13.75
Attending Physicians	75.63	24.38
Oncologists	76.25	23.75

Table 3. GEOGRAPHICAL LOCATION OF DOCTORS

Physicians	Area	
	North %	Center+South %
Family Doctors	34.03	31.72
Attending Physicians	39.10	20.00
Oncologists	26.87	48.28

In Tables 1, 2 and 3, some personal and geographical particulars of the sample of physicians are reported. It can be noticed how the greater part of the physicians who completed our questionnaire (54.58%) are from an age range of 31 to 40 (almost 50% of the sample, against approximately 30% over 41 years and 20% below 30 years).

In evaluating tendencies of the physicians on the above defined areas, we sought to differentiate the effect of the variable 'type of activity' and age, forming two sub-groups.

The first group consisted of physicians carrying out the same activity but of different age, while the second group consisted of physicians in the same age range but operating in different fields. The results obtained, reported in the contingency tables show that the greatest number of statistically important differences were due to the different professional environments rather than age. This datum confirms what is maintained by various research studies already referred to on the effect of professional experience on attitudes.

As regard sex, we find respectively a prevalence of men over women which does in fact reflect the distribution by sex in the medical population. As far as geographic origin is concerned, the major part of responses were obtained in the north of Italy, compared to the Centre-South. The significance of this is probably to be found in practical reasons as well as in interpretations of a sociological nature which we did not analyse and on which we will consequently pass no comment.

Table 4 shows the single statements of our questionnaire as they were grouped by us into the 5 attitude groups described earlier. We should like to point out that in evaluating the data, the responses to some items were inverted in order to maintain a single direction of attitude.

The statements requiring this kind of inverted evaluation are indicated on Table 4 by an asterisk. (*) In Tables 5,6,7,8 and 9, the distribution of the responses in percentages for each single attitude and for each 'type of activity' are reported, as well as the X2 values for each cross comparison performed. The X2 value for group 1 is as a whole very significant (p < .001).

For reasons of brevity only certain of the histograms relative to the first attitude group are enclosed here, that is, the group relative to the information the physician should or should not give to the patient and his/her family regarding diagnosis, prognosis and therapy in the terminal phase.

Table 4. ATTITUDES TOWARDS DUTY TO INFORM OR NOT A PATIENT ON DIAGNOSIS, PROGNOSIS AND THERAPY
A

7   As cancer is already difficult enough to treat, the risk of having to deal with a depressed patient, having informed him or her on the diagnosis, should be avoided.

8   The patient's negative reactions, on knowing he or she has cancer usually go beyond the advantage of being informed.

13 It is better not to use the word 'cancer' when a patient asks about his or her condition.

19* Patients in the terminal phase of illness should be informed, to prepare themselves spiritually for death.

35 In the terminal phase of the illness, most doctors would rather not talk about the patients' diagnoses, even when expressely requested by the patients.

44 It is usually better to discuss with a member of his or her family what to communicate to the cancer patient.

47 The patient should be informed on his or her diagnosis and illness as soon as this is assessed.

48 Patients have the right to take part in the planning of their therapy.

49 Patients and their families have the right to have full knowledge of the diagnosis of their illness.

51 Patients should be informed on their prognosis even when unfavourable.

52 When the prognosis is unfavourable, doctors prefer to inform members of the family rather than the patient.

(continued)

Table 4. (Continued)

ATTITUDES OF PHYSICIANS TOWARDS PERFORMING OR NOT AGGRESSIVE
THERAPY

B

3   It is important to ensure that the terminally ill patient has a peaceful
    atmosphere and a dignified death rather than fight it out until the end.

4   Patients affected by those types of cancer, for which the 5-year survival
    rate is low, - e.g. cancer of the oesophagus, stomach, lung, pancreas -
    have no benefit from aggressive therapy.

14 Most oncological therapy adopted for patients affected by cancer in an
    advanced phase, cause complications, pain and expenses with no actual
    benefit for the patients.

15 Therapy to stop cancer evolution should always be attempted as long as
    the patient is alive, not withstanding possible serious side effects.

16 Radical surgery of cancer is rarely advisable for patients over 70 years
    old.

17 Patients affected by cancer of the prostate benefit from oestrogen
    therapy to such as extent that possible complications should be over-
    looked.

27 Patients have the right to take any type of drug, in order to relieve
    pain.

28 Aggressive therapy should be used more readily with young patients than
    with old patients.

33 Doctors should prolong the patient's life as much as possible, by what-
    ever means, even if suffering is prolonged consequently.

39 Aggressive therapy should be used more readily with working or socially
    active patients than with non-working or socially isolated patients.

45 Patients who passively follow therapy directions can be treated better.

ATTITUDES OF PHYSICIANS TOWARDS PATIENTS' RESOURCES FACE-TO-FACE
WITH CANCER

C

2   Being given an uncertain prognosis is distressing for the patient.

5   Experience shows that, since those patients affected by cancer, who wish
    to be informed on their illness, have negative reactions on knowing about
    it, they do not actually want to know that they have cancer.

9   Patients would suffer from an irreversible psychological shock if they
    knew that their cancer cannot be cured.

10* The patient who is affected by cancer can be considered lucky in having
    the time to prepare himself or herself for death, rather than facing it
    abruptly.

11 The hope of recovering can make the patient feel better.

26 Men can withstand being diagnosed for cancer better than women.

34 Male patients cooperate more than female patients.

37 Cancer patients in general should not be informed of the gravity of their illness.

58 Cancer patients prefer to be treated by a specialist than by a family doctor.

ATTITUDE TOWARDS DEATH

D

1 Men can accept belief in nonexistence after death.

6 No man can maintain a state of mental welfare knowing he or she is going to die soon.

18* The immortality of a person consists of the memory he or she leaves behind through material goods, examples from his or her life, reputation or children.

20* Detaching himself or herself from the things of this world, a person can have a truer or closer relationship with others and be ready for death.

21 A person ought to live without the knowledge that one day he or she would die.

22* To be a realist, a man should accept that he cannot exist after death.

23 It is often more tragic to have cancer at 20 than at an older age.

30* Usually elderly patients find it easier to face death than younger patients.

36 Patients should always be encouraged not to lose hope.

ATTITUDE TOWARDS THE ASSUMPTION OR NOT OF RESPONSIBILITIES TO THE PATIENT AND DYING PERSON ON THE PART OF THE FAMILIES, SOCIETY AND PHYSICIAN

E

12 One should avoid dealing directly with the feelings of a patient towards death.

24 If a patient refuses to follow medical advice, it is better to pass him or her onto another colleague.

25 Patients should be convinced to follow our therapy.

29 Patients should be dissuaded from dying at home, owing to the burden this would cause the family.

31 Sometimes doctors and hospital staff tend to 'get rid of' patients in their terminal phase.

(continued)

Table 4. (Continued)

32 It is easier to treat a married patient, rather than an unmarried patient, due to the help provided by the family.

38 A psychological and/or social evaluation should play an integral part in the initial assessment of the cancer patient's needs.

39 Aggressive therapy should be used more readily with working or socially active patients than with non-working or socially isolated patients.

40 Doctors consider the death of a patient as a personal defeat.

41 The patient is often ostracized by his or her family and friends.

42 Doctors tend to be interested in illness rather than the patient as a person.

43 Doctors tend to be less understanding with patients affected by a type of personal responsibility-linked cancer, (e.g. Bronchial cancer and tobacco) than with those affected by other types of cancer.

46 Doctors should avoid any emotional involvement with cancer patients.

50 The psycho-social aspects of cancer ought to be dealt with by mental health specialists as well.

53 Society should bear the economic burden of terminally ill patients.

54 Doctors should bear in mind the sexual needs of cancer patients.

55 It is better to share the burden of one cancer patient with other colleagues, rather than take on the total responsibility of his or her course of treatment.

56 The anxiety which terminally ill patients can transmit is sometimes unbearable.

57 The family of a cancer patient should be aware that a terminally ill patient should have the possibility of dying at home.

59 Non-hospitalized terminally ill patient should be assisted by the family doctor rather than a specialist.

60 Treatment at home is more comfortable for the patient.

61 Family doctors should be more fully informed on cancer therapy.

62 Since a family doctor is not a specialist, if one of his or her patients dies of cancer, his or her moral burden is greater.

Table 5. ATTITUDES TOWARD THE PHYSICIAN'S DUTY TO INFORM OR NOT A PATIENT ON DIAGNOSIS, PROGNOSIS AND THERAPY

	Fam.Doctors n.160 %	Att.Phys. n.160 %	Oncologists n.160 %	Total n.480 %
True	51.93	46.70	43.41	47.35
False	32.78	37.44	40.28	36.84
Unknown	13.86	15.51	14.03	14.47
No ans.	1.42	.34	2.27	1.34

	Fam.Dr./Att.Phys.	X^2=29.202 df.1 p<.001 (true vs false)
	Fam.Dr./Oncol.	X^2=26.850 df.1 p<.001 (true vs false)
	Fam.Dr./Oncol.	X^2= 4.744 df.1 p<.05 (true vs false)

Table 6. ATTITUDES OF PHYSICIANS TOWARDS PERFORMING OR NOT AGGRESSIVE
THERAPY ON PATIENTS

	Family Doctor			Attending Physician			Oncologist			Total		
	No.	%	%	No.	%	%	No.	%	%	No.	%	%
True 1-1	733	50.90	32.62	767	53.26	34.13	747	51.78	33.24	2247	52.01	100.0
False 2-2	488	33.89	34.91	405	28.13	28.97	505	35.07	36.01	1398	32.36	100.0
Unknown 3-3	203	14.10	32.27	256	17.78	40.70	170	11.81	27.03	629	14.56	100.0
No Answer 9-9	16	1.11	34.78	12	.83	26.09	18	1.25	39.13	46	1.06	100.0
Total	1440	100.0	33.33	1440	100.0	33.33	1440	100.0	33.33	4320	100.0	100.0

Fam.Dr./Att.Phys. X^2= 7.485 df=1 p<.01 (true and false)

Fam.Dr./Att.Phys. X^2=13.175 df=1 p<.001 (false and unknown)

Att.Phys./Oncol. X^2= 8.622 df=1 p<.01 (true and false)

Att.Phys./Oncol. X^2=11.869 df=1 p<.001 (true and unknown)

Table 7. ATTITUDES OF PHYSICIANS TOWARDS PATIENTS' RESOURCES FACE-TO-FACE
WITH CANCER

	Family Doctor			Attending Physician			Oncologist			Total		
	No.	%	%	No.	%	%	No.	%	%	No.	%	%
True 1-1	858	59.58	33.36	823	57.15	32.00	891	61.88	34.64	2572	59.54	100.0
False 2-3	317	22.01	34.05	304	21.11	32.65	310	21.53	33.30	931	21.55	100.0
Unknown 3-3	250	17.36	32.13	304	21.11	39.07	224	15.56	28.79	778	18.01	100.0
No Answer 9-9	15	1.04	38.46	9	.63	23.08	15	1.04	38.46	39	.90	100.0
Total	1440	100.0	33.33	1440	100.0	33.33	1440	100.0	33.33	4320	100.0	100.0

Fam.Dr./Att.Phys. X^2= 5.831 df=1 p<.02 (true vs unknown)

Att.Phys./Oncol. X^2= 7.416 df=1 p<.01 (false vs unknown)

Att.Phys./Oncol. X^2=14.755 df=1 p<.001 (true vs unknown)

Table 8. ATTITUDES OF PHYSICIANS TOWARDS DEATH

	Family Doctor			Attending Physician			Oncologist			Total		
	No.	%	%	No.	%	%	No.	%	%	No.	%	%
True 1-1	504	35.00	34.19	484	33.61	32.84	486	33.75	32.97	1474	34.12	100.0
False 2-2	725	50.35	33.36	743	51.60	34.19	705	48.96	32.44	2173	50.30	100.0
Unknown 3-3	183	12.71	30.15	195	13.54	32.13	229	15.90	37.73	607	14.05	100.0
No Answer 9-9	28	1.94	42.42	18	1.25	27.27	20	1.39	30.30	66	1.53	100.0
Total	1440	100.0	33.33	1440	100.0	33.33	1440	100.0	33.33	4320	100.0	100.0

Fam.Dr./Oncol. X^2=5.050 fd=1 p<.02 (false vs unknown)

Fam.Dr./Oncol. X^2=4.906 fd=1 p<.05 (true vs unknown)

Table 9. ATTITUDE TOWARDS THE ASSUMPTION OR NOT OF RESPONSIBILITIES TO THE PATIENT AND DYING PERSON ON THE PART OF FAMILIES, SOCIETY AND THE PHYSICIAN

	Family Doctor			Attending Physician			Oncologist			Total		
	No.	%	%	No.	%	%	No.	%	%	No.	%	%
True 1-1	2195	57.16	33.12	2267	59.04	34.21	2165	56.38	32.67	6627	57.53	100.0
False 2-2	1216	31.67	34.61	1126	29.32	32.05	1171	30.49	33.33	3513	30.49	100.0
Unknown 3-3	375	9.77	31.07	435	11.33	36.04	397	10.34	32.89	1207	10.48	100.0
No Answer 9-9	54	1.41	31.21	12	.31	6.94	107	2.79	61.85	173	1.50	100.0
Total	3840	100.0	33.33	3840	100.0	33.33	3840	100.0	33.33	11520	100.	100.0

Fam.Dr./Att.Phys. X^2=4.573 fd=1 p<.05 (true vs false)

Fam.Dr./Att.Phys. X^2=7.618 fd=1 p<.01 (false vs unknown)

DISCUSSION

The initial hypothesis which tended to look for differences of opinion or attitude deriving from differences in professionality, is confirmed by data inherent in the first scale (attitudes towards informing) in a statistically important way (X global mean: p<.001). This significance is not, however, maintained for the other 4 scales but only for some of the items contained in them. Given the extent of the study, we shall present only some of the important results which are particularly relevant to the topic we are dealing with here.

A preliminary word should be said on the differences we expected : although they are more or less verified as tendencies, they are not such as to state that different attitudes correspond (or are determined by) differences in role.

In particular, we can notice that as regards the image of man, of his resources, of death, of its real inacceptability and of the psychological and social necessity of taking on the responsibility of the patient's well-being in the terminal phase, as well as opinions on the psycho-physical toll and the applicability of aggressive therapies, all three categories are on average in line.

The data on informing, on the other hand, shows absolute disharmony. We can examine at least 3 components which determine the informative choice and are weighed differently for the different professions:

- compliance with norms (inform because so required by the praxes of clinical research)
- exigencies of clarity (inform to obtain patient's long term collaboration in complex therapy)
- exigencies of peace (self/illness/feeling good relationship (inform because it is the right thing to do)

These three components of the necessity of informing are placed in relation to response belonging to different scales.

The scale concerning informing consists of 11 items - statements. The direction in which they are read (except for the inverted ones marked *) is that the response TRUE confirms a statement on NOT giving information.

We can use the statement categorization scheme:

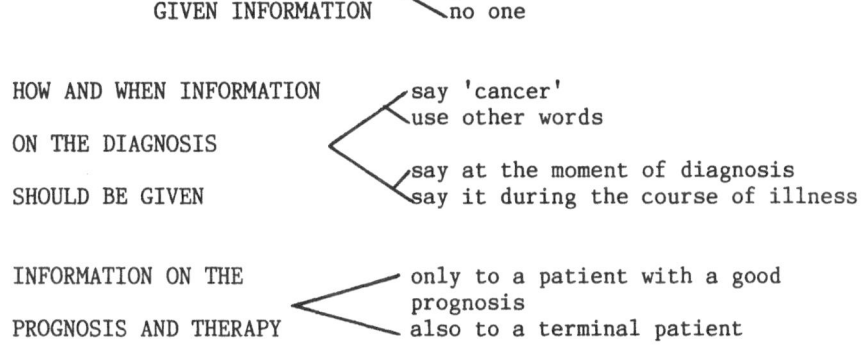

Let us now examine some results that show that there are very discriminating differences between assuming the 'DON'T TELL' position for each category and each response.

As can be seen from Table 5, family doctors inform less than attending physicians who, in turn, inform less than oncologists with statistically significant differences. ($p < .001$). The differences in the non-choices, which we can find reported in the histograms, are also interesting.

The need to inform is evidently greater for oncologists who from the point of view of a therapeutic role require greater collaboration on the part of the patient and as a scientific reference, are more influenced by an atmosphere which in the Latin world is often defined 'Anglosaxon' in which recognition of the duty to inform, awareness of the patient is often considered an 'a priori' as regards the doctor-patient relationship when such informative praxis is actually not juridically standard. Hence the oncologist 'should' and 'can' tell (he is supposed to tell). This practice does, however, vacillate in the relationship with the terminally ill. The questions regarding the latter (35.19.51) do in fact show a difficulty in choosing true or false, particularly for oncologists. The death of the patient is a levelling element on this scale, too, where, moreover, significant differences emerge. For everyone, in fact, the patient in the terminal phase must not be given the diagnosis even when he expressly requests it and nor must he be informed of an unfavourable prognosis; it is not certain whether or not it is important for a patient to be able to prepare him or herself to face death. We shall have a better look at the differences of opinion on this subject.

Still on the subject of informing, we would like to emphasize that there is general agreement on talking to the family rather than the patient. Oncologists, however, prefer not to discuss it first with members of the patient's family, but rather with the patient, contrary to physicians in other professional fields. (item 44)

Standard praxis as per the Medical Deontological Codex and Italian legislation are quite ambiguous in that the patient must give his or her consent to therapy, but the ways and means of making him or her aware are no better defined; art.30 Italian deontological codex states: "a serious or unfavourable prognosis may be kept hidden from the patient, but not from his family. In all cases, however, the patients' will, freely expressed, must constitute an element which determines the physician's behaviour".

Physicians are thus in line with what is juridically defined. This is true to a greater extent of oncologists who, compared to family doctors, due to the nature and practice of their research, make more use in the application of the formulae of informed consent. Although it is not our concern here to open a discussion on legislative ambiguities, we do, however, consider it useful to point out that from the results of our study, certain figures emerge. One, the oncologist, adheres more readily to the norms, another is identifiable with the doctor - good person stereotype, who cares about the needs of his patient but who believes it correct not to use the word 'cancer' (71,88%) and to keep information to himself and to decide when it is or it is not the right moment to pass the information on - the family doctor. A third figure, the attending physician, seems to suffer particularly from a lack of reference points regarding his professional identity face-to-face with the oncology patient. The greatest number of contradictions emerge for the third figure, that of the attending physician. These contradictions are between certain statements and those items which refer to the professional category as something abstract (e.g. "usually, doctors").

The need to be kind, gentle and reassuring for patients is at the same time accompanied by the emergence of an abstract figure of doctor who tends to keep his distance from the terminally ill patient (item 31 , true for 71% of attending physicians) and above all are more concerned with treating the illness and not the patient (item 42, true for 61% of attending physicians).

Let us now examine some responses to statements concerning assisting terminally ill patients contained in other attitude groups. As the most general difference, we should like to emphasize that the oncologist is the least inclined to pass a negative judgment on the patient knowing the diagnosis and prognosis of the illness (item 9-5); family doctors are more undecided as to whether or not the terminal patient ought to ask for or receive information regarding his situation. For everyone, it emerges that men should live in the awareness that one day they will die (item 21) but it is not the doctor's task to tell them to prepare themselves for that day.

The implication that the death of the patient is a defeat for the doctor is rejected more than accepted, although there is, on the whole, general agreement (item 40). Item 54 according to which the anxiety trans-

mitted by a dying person could be unbearable is again underlined in oncologists (50% true) who become the most emotionally involved in this relationship. The personal and professional consequences are certainly manifold.
On average, only 28% of our overall sample do, however, maintain that
emotional involvement should be avoided. As regards home treatment, everyone
maintains that it is more comfortable for terminally ill patients (mean 77%),
but here diverse images of the patient emerge: 41% of oncologists maintain
that the patient prefers to be treated by a specialist; attending physicians
are uncertain (50%), and family doctors maintain that the patient prefers to
be treated by them (item 58). Furthermore, when the terminally ill patient
is not hospitalized, oncologists alone believe that he should be assisted by
a specialist.

Divergent interpretations thus emerge regarding professional duties
(oncologists, for example, believe that family doctors ought to be better
informed on oncological therapies than the latter believe) (item 61), as well
as for doctor – patient relationships. All the professional categories are
afraid of losing compliance but, as we have seen, the informative praxis is
different for each of the 3 groups of physicians. Analysis of item 56 provides another important piece of data. Oncologists seem to be the category
that suffers most from the unbearable anxiety that the terminally ill patient
may transmit and which surrounds him. (Item 56 was true for 59% of the
oncologists against 46% of the attending physicians and 47% of the family
doctors).

An interpretation could place this more highly changed emotional aspect
in relation to the type of rapport which is set up between the oncologist
and the patient: greater availability, more open-ness and greater frankness.
It is not for us here to go into depth on the subject of the value of re-
lationship/cost, doctor/patient benefit, but rather we should like to
emphasize the necessity of a suitable formative procedure that begins in the
university environment and then continues on a permanent basis, manifesting
itself in the objectives and work methodologies in the reality of all medical
activities.

ACKNOWLEDGEMENT

This research was realised by the contribution of the Ministry of Health,
Italy.

REFERENCES

Baanson, C. B. 1975, Psychologic and emotional issues in cancer: the
    psychotherapeutic care of cancer patients, Semin Oncol., 2:293–30.
Blanchard, G.C.,1981, Attitude towards cancer: the impact of a comprehen-
    sive oncology course on the second year medical students, Cancer,
    47:2756–2762.
Brim, O.G., Freeman, H. E., Levine, S. and Scotch, N.A., 1970, "The Dying
    Patient", Russell Sage Foundation, New York.
Glaser, B.G. and Strauss, A. L., 1965, "Awareness of Dying", Aldine, Chicago.
Hays, M. D., 1985, Effects of intensive clinical exposure on attitudes of
    medical students towards cancer related problems, Cancer, 55:636–642.
Hoerni, B. and Lagarde, C., 1983, Attitudes de medecins et des etudiantes
    en medecine vis-a-vis des cancers et des cancereux, Bull.Cancer, 705:
    394–400.
Holland, J. F., 1973, Psychological Aspects of Cancer, in "Cancer Medicine",
    J.F. Holland and E. Frei eds., Lea and Febeiger, Philadelphia.
Krant, M. J., 1976, Problems of the Physician in Presenting the Patient with
    the diagnosis, in "Cancer: the Behavioural Dimension". Cullen, ed.,
    Raven Press, New York.

Ley, P., 1977, Psychological Studies of Doctor Patient Communication, in
   "Medical Psychology, Vol. I", S Rachman, ed., Pergamon Press, Oxford.
Novak, H. D., 1979, Changes in physicians' attitudes towards telling the
   cancer patient, J.A.M.A., 2 241 9:897–900.
Poole, A. D. and Sanson-Fisher, R. W., 1979, Understanding the patient:
   a neglected aspect of medical education, Soc. Sci. Med., 13a:37–43.
Reise, R. S., 1983, "La Medicina e il Regno della Technologia",
   Feltrinelli, Mi.
Reynolds, P. M., Sanson-Fisher, R. W., Desmond-Poole, A., Harker, J. and
   Byrne, M. J., Cancer and communication: information giving in an
   oncology clinic, Br. Med. Journ., 282:1449–1451.

A COMPARISON OF FOUR OUTCOME MEASURES OF TERMINAL CARE

Irene Higginson, Angela Wade and Mark McCarthy

Department of Community Medicine
University College of London
London, U.K.

In the United Kingdom and Republic of Ireland there are now over 170 terminal care support services operating from hospices, hospitals or the community (St Christophers, 1987). The services, usually teams, follow the hospice philosophy in caring for terminally ill cancer patients and families. More teams are planned or are being developed, in some areas expanding the service to include terminally ill patients other than those diagnosed as suffering from cancer. There is a need to evaluate these teams and to seek ways to improve care, but who should make the assessments of their work and how should these assessments be made?

Most units collect data on aspects of their process of care, such as number of patients seen, number of home visits, drugs used, duration of survival (St Joseph's, 1986) and use this in annual reports which are often geared towards raising awareness or fund-raising. However, in terminal care there are no agreed standards of 'good' process of care, and units disagree on ideal policies for visiting and case load (Ward, 1987). Therefore this cannot reliably inform us about the outcome of care.

Often the evaluation of the outcome of health care relies on measures of mortality and morbidity. In terminal care these are clearly not appropriate. A variety of different scales and forms of assessment have been used. Existing studies have often concentrated on the management of symptoms, commonly pain (Parkes, 1985) or the place of care and death (Parkes, 1980) or patient or family anxiety (Parkes, 1985). In some instances satisfaction with care and cost have been reported (Parkes, 1980). To achieve an assessment of 'quality of life' more global scales have been used, but these are usually concerned with the patient's needs. However, the hospice movement seeks not only to serve the needs of the patient but also those of the family (Saunders, 1978). In addition, support teams also deal with the provision of services and financial benefits (Garfield, 1978; Bloomsbury Support Team). Any scales designed to evaluate support teams fully need to take all these objectives into account. Mount and Scott (1983) observed that the outcome of hospice care is often not reflected by existing measures.

Taking assessments directly from patients is often difficult; the patients are ill and may die before they can be identified or contacted. This has lead to studies based on the views of bereaved spouses (Parkes, 1980). However, although the spouse can inform us about his/her own views and needs, the assessment will be affected by his/her own grieving process. In addition, assessment is naturally limited to patients with spouses or close family. An alternative is to use the assessments of the health professionals, but do these represent the patient's view?

In a current study we are looking at the correlation between four different methods of assessing the work of a support team: a locally developed system of internal audit used by the team to monitor care and predict difficult cases, a quality of life index, assessments from patients and assessments made by the patient's family (nearest carer). This paper reports the early comparisons of the support team's and the families assessments with the patients' views of care; data collection is still continuing.

PATIENTS AND METHODS

Data was collected over a six month period from February to August 1987. The assessments were made on patients and their families (in all cases 'family' refers to the patient's nearest carer, usually spouse) receiving home care from a terminal care support team (Bloomsbury Support Team, 1987; Evans and McCarthy, 1984) based in Bloomsbury district. This is a central London health district with a population of 120,000 people. The team is multidisciplinary, consisting of 2 nursing sisters, a social worker, a part-time doctor, and administrator/secretary and a consultant radiotherapist officially in charge. They offer advice and support for terminally ill cancer patients within the district; clinical responsibility remains with the referring hospital consultant or general practitioner while the team provide professional advice, co-ordination of services including practical and financial needs, and support for the patient, family and professional carers. A 24 hour on-call service is provided. Much of the work is domiciliary and the team has no in-patient beds specifically for their patients.

Two of the outcome measures rely on assessments made by the members of the support team. Patients and carers were assessed at referral, then weekly until death, according to an audit schedule and a quality of life index. For internal audit the Support Team Assessment Schedule (STAS) was used (McCarthy). This schedule has sixteen items: aspects directly concerned with the patient and family, including symptom control, anxiety, insight, communication and planning; and aspects concerned with the services, including practical and financial needs, communication between professionals and the support and advice needed for other professionals. It is based on the team's goals of care. Each item is graded on a five point scale (0-4) and there are definitions for the score level of each item. A high score indicates severe problems. The definitions for an example item, patient anxiety, are shown in Table 1. The scores are recorded weekly on all patients in care, from referral to discharge or death. In addition the team makes a weekly record of the patient's current location and the contact with the team.

The quality of life scale used is HRCA - Quality of Life index (a modified form of Spitzer QL-index) previously used in the United States National Hospice Study. This scale has five components: mobility, daily living, health, support and outlook. Each component is measured on a three point scale and a patient's total score can range from 0 (worst) to 10 (best). (This is in the opposite direction to STAS.) The original scale was used in pretests and validation tests by more than 150 physicians to rate 879 patients and showed significant correlations between the scores of health professionals and patients. The modification made in the National Hospice Study consisted of substituting the item 'Activity' for a new item not based on working activities 'Mobility'.

Table 1. DEFINITIONS OF THE SCORES FOR THE ITEM 'PATIENT ANXIETY'

<u>Definition</u> = Effect of his/her anxiety on the patient

0 = None

1 = Worry over changes. No physical or behavioural symptoms
of anxiety. Concentration not affected.

2 = Waiting for changes or problems. Occasional physical or
behavioural symptoms of anxiety. Concentration affected
but still possible at times.

3 = Anxious often. Physical/behavioural symptoms. Concentration markedly affected.

4 = Completely and continuously preoccupied with anxiety and
worries. Unable to think of other matters.

Lastly, an external researcher approached the referred patients and asked for an interview. The initial introduction was made by a support team member and followed up by a telephone call or letter. Each patient and his or her family were visited at home and asked separately to assess six schedule items which the patient and family could practically score themselves; symptom control, patient anxiety, family anxiety, wasted time, need for practical aids, communication between professionals and the patient and family. For each item the patient and family were given the standard definitions used in the schedule and asked to score themselves on the scale describing the last week. They were also asked to comment in open questions on the various services, their worries and anxieties and on their needs. The single interview scores were matched with the support team scores in the same time period. Where possible the interviews were conducted by two interviewers simultaneously with the patient and family in separate rooms.

The mean scores are presented (with associated 95% confidence intervals); two sample t-tests are used to test for differences between groups. Spearman Rank and Pearson correlations have been applied to test for associations between the scores. Significance level is taken at 5% ($p < 0.05$), two tailed test.

RESULTS

We present here the preliminary results of the comparisons between the support team's assessments and those of the family and the patient's own assessments.

Of 64 patients referred to the team during the study period, 55 were receiving home care at some time (the remainder were primarily hospital inpatients or were transferred to hospice care almost immediately). Records on the terminal care schedule and the HRCA QL index and the Karnofsky index were made on all 55 patients. Home interviews were achieved for 32 (58%) patients. Failures to interview include; 5 patients who refused contact from either an interviewer or would only accept limited contact from the support team, 12 who died before they could be seen, 1 patient who was suffering from senile dementia and 2 from depression and were not interviewed, and 3 cases where the support team felt unable to ask for interview.

207

Table 2. MEAN SCORES OF THE PATIENTS, FAMILIES AND TEAMS

	Patient			Family			Team		
	N	Mean Score	95% Confidence Interval Upper Limit	N	Mean Score	95% Confidence Interval Upper Limit	N	Mean Score	95% Confidence Interval Upper Limit
Symptom control	25	1.80	2.21	25	2.36+	2.75	32	1.41	1.71
Patient anxiety	27	0.96	1.42	25	1.72+	2.31	32	1.45	1.76
Family anxiety	24	2.13	2.60	26	1.92	2.36	30	1.73*	2.01
Practical aids	27	0.15	0.29	28	0.11	0.23	32	0.31	0.58
Wastes time	28	0.07	0.22	28	0.14	0.32	32	0.06	0.19
Communication from professionals to patient and family	26	0.08	0.24	28	0.26	0.60	32	0.47*	0.76

Compared to patients scores, two sample t-test: * $p < 0.05$
+ borderline $p < 0.1$

Table 3. CORRELATION OF FAMILY AND TEAM SCORES WITH PATIENTS SCORES:
TOTAL SCORES FROM ITEMS, SYMPTOM CONTROL AND PATIENT AND
FAMILY ANXIETY

	Number	Spearman Correlation rho	Pearson Correlation r
Family	15	0.486+	0.406
Support team	26	0.400*	0.532**

** p < 0.005   * p < 0.05   + borderline p < 0.1

Of the 32 patients visited, 4 did not have family (nearest carers) who
could be interviewed. Of the 28 families interviewed, 24 (86% were the
patient's spouse, the other 4 were living with and caring for the patient.
8 patients and 5 families missed one or more assessments on the form.
Patients failed to complete if they were very ill; families were sometimes
reluctant to assess their own or the patient's anxiety and in 2 cases there
were language difficulties. The average time for interview was 30 minutes.

The mean scores for the patients, families and support team are shown
in Table 2. The numbers are small so we have concentrated on looking for
trends in the data rather than absolute tests. For symptom control the
support team tend to score lower (less problems) than the patients and the
family to score higher (more problems). In assessing patient anxiety there
is a tendency for the patients to score lower than both the support team
and the family. None of these differences are statistically significant at
the 5% level. There is a significant difference between the support team
assessments and the patients' assessments of the families' anxiety, where
the team score lower.

The scores for the 3 service items are generally lower (many scored 0)
indicating less need, and the mean scores are similar in all groups. The
support team score higher for communication from professionals to patient
and family, implying they identify problems when the patient does not.

The scores for patient anxiety, symptom control and family anxiety have
been totalled for the patient, the family and the support team. Cases where
complete totals could not be calculated due to the score for one or more
items being missed have been excluded from this preliminary analysis. Table
3 shows the correlation coefficients testing for associations between the
total scores in these cases. In only one case did the family's total score
agree exactly with the patients total score, in 8 cases the scores were
higher and in 6 cases the scores were lower. (The differences between family
and patients total scores ranged from +9 to -3.) No significant associations
were shown at the 5% level although it should be noted that only 15 cases
could be compared.

In 8 cases the team's total scores agreed exactly with the patients'
totals, in 11 cases the scores were lower, in 7 the scores were higher.
(The differences between team and patients total scores ranged from +3 to
-5.) Significant correlations were found with Spearman Rank and Pearson
correlations (p < 0.05 and p < 0.005, respectively).

DISCUSSION

Taking assessments on the outcome of care directly from patients has been criticised for two reasons. In some instances it is considered an intrusion. In our study most patients were willing to help, except for a few who did not want contact from any source. However, they were only visited once and might have found repeated assessments intrusive. A more serious difficulty is the reliability and completeness of assessments from severely ill patients. In two recent studies of patients in hospice and home care settings only one half to one third of patients in care survived until or were well enough to be interviewed (Ward, 1985; Lunt, 1986). Our study where only 58% of patients could be interviewed supports these findings. If the most ill patients therefore cannot be assessed by interview this is a potential source of bias.

Assessments by family members may be affected in unknown ways by the families' own process of grief. Only a few very recent studies have considered this. Ahmetzai comparing the assessments of relatives and close friends in the bereavement period showed that these did not correlate with self-assessments of patients during their life. The assessments are also influenced by the place of care and the family may be more aware (Parkes, 1985) or over report symptoms when patients are at home. Our findings are compatible with this interpretation. When families' assessments are used these should be considered as measuring, at least in part, the families' 'pain', 'anxiety' etc. and not the patients'.

We have developed the Support Team Assessment Schedule (STAS) for terminal care support teams to assess their work. The assessments are easy and quick to make and are incorporated into the team's routine work. Data is complete and collected on all patients throughout care: this allows care to be monitored and for the results to be fedback to the teams quickly. However, the inherent problem of self audit is that it relies on the assessments of the professionals involved in care, who may be inclined to assess their own work favourably and give scores which do not reflect the patient's view. The preliminary results of this study indicate that the support team's assessments do correlate with the patients scores. We found, however, that there is a tendency for the team to rate symptom control as less of a problem, and patient anxiety as more of a problem, than the patient's self-rating. As the data collection is continuing more accurate analysis will become available and the comparisons using other measures will be made.

Although significant, none of the correlation coefficients reported here indicate strong linear associations, so we can not assume that one assessment is exactly represented by another. Dying is often a private and personal process experienced differently by the patient, who undergoes it, the relative who grieves, and the professionals. There is no absolute measure of 'good' dying or terminal care to choose as a criterion for validation. The STAS has a utility as a convenient method for teams to audit their work which gives a representation of the patient's view. However, each assessor, patient, family and support team may be giving different view points, each appropriate and valid.

ACKNOWLEDGEMENTS

We are grateful to 'Help the Hospices' for funding this research. We thank the members of the Bloomsbury Support Team: Patrick Dixon, Jill Highet, Julia Franklin, Margaret Vincent, Joyce Bell and Jeffrey Tobias for their careful thought given to this study; members of the Bloomsbury District Department of Community Medicine for their contribution to the study; Pamela Sokel (volunteer) and Debbie Atkinson (medical student) for assisting in the interviews and the patients and families for giving up their valuable time to see us.

REFERENCES

Bloomsbury Support Team, 1987, Home and ward care, National Temperance Hospital, London.

Evans, C. and McCarthy, M., 1984, Referral and Survival of patients accepted by a terminal care support team, Journal of Epidemiology and Community Health, 38:310-4.

Garfield, C., 1978, "Psychosocial Care of the Dying Patient", McGraw-Hill, New York.

Lunt, B. J., 1986, The assessment of symptoms and mood in terminally ill cancer patients (Abstract): in "Psychosocial Issues in Malignant Disease",M. Watson and S. Greer, eds., Pergamon, London.

McCarthy, M. and Higginson, I., Self audit in terminal care, in preparation.

Mount, B. M. and Scott, J. F., 1983, Whither hospice evaluation? Journal of Chronic Disease; 36:731-6.

Parkes, C. M., 1980, Terminal care: evaluation of an advisory domiciliary service at St. Christopher's Hospice, Postgraduate Medical Journal, 56:685-9.

Parkes, C. M., 1985, Terminal care: home, hospital or hospice? Lancet, i:155-7.

Saunders, C. M., 1978, in "The Management of Terminal Disease", C.M. Saunders ed., Edward Arnold, London.

St. Christopher's Hospice Information Service, 1987, Directory of Hospice Services, St. Christopher's Hospice, London.

St. Joseph's Hospice Annual Report, 1986, St. Joseph's Hospice, London.

Ward, A. W. M., 1985, Home care services for the terminally ill: a report for the Nuffield Foundation, Medical Care Research Unit, Department of Community Medicine, University of Sheffield.

Ward, A. W. M., 1987, Home care services - an alternative to hospices? Community Medicine, 9(1):47-54.

CONTRIBUTORS

J. Beckmann	Clinical Psychology Department, Odense University Hospital, Odense, Denmark
M. Bond	Department of Psychological Medicine, University of Glasgow, Scotland, U.K.
A. Bowling	Department of General Practice, St. Bartholomews Hospital Medical College, London, England, U.K.
E. Brewis	Nursing Administration, Royal Hospital for Sick Children, Glasgow, Scotland, U.K.
F. Campione	Dipartimento di Pscicolgia, Universita Degli Studi di Bologna, Bologna, Italy
F. Cianfriglia	Department of Psychology, Istituto Tumori, Genova, Italy
A. Couldrick	Sir Michael Sobell House, Churchill Hospital, Oxford, England, U.K.
N. Crotti	Department of Psychology, Istituto Tumori, Genova, Italy
E. De Bruin	Department of Pediatrics, University Hospital Groningen, Groningen, The Netherlands
F. Delfalco	Department of Psychology, Istituto Tumori, Genova, Italy
N. Delvaux	Department of Psychology, Centre D'Aides aux Mourants, Bruxelles, Belgium
C. Farvacques	Department of Psychology, Centre D'Aides aux Mourants, Bruxelles, Belgium
R. Feinmann	Stepping Hill Hospital, Stockport, England, U.K.
P. Floriet	JALMALV, Grenoble, France
D. Frampton	St. Joseph's Hospice, London, England, U.K.
S. Frierdich	University of Wisconsin Hospital and Clinics, Wisconsin, U.S.A.

A. Gilmore	Prince and Princess of Wales Hospice, Glasgow, Scotland, U.K.
S. Gilmore	Department of Continuing Education, Stirling University, Scotland, U.K.
F. Gunz	Department of Clinical Oncology, Royal North Shore Hospital, St Leonards, Australia
I. Higginson	Department of Community Medicine, London, England, U.K.
G.B. Humphrey	Department of Pediatrics, University Hospital Groningen, Groningen, The Netherlands
R. Illsley	Age Concern Research Europe, University of Bath, Bath, England, U.K.
K. Inoue	Department of Psychology, Tokyo Metropolitan Institute of Gerontology, Tokyo, Japan
N. James	Institute of Health Care Studies, University College of Swansea, Swansea, England, U.K.
M. Jolley	PLUS Self Help Association, Edinburgh, Scotland, U.K.
W.A. Kamps	Department of Pediatrics, University Hospital Groningen, Groningen, The Netherlands
R. Kastenbaum	Adult Development and Aging Program, Arizona State University, Arizona, U.S.A.
A. Kingma	Department of Pediatrics, University Hospital Groningen, Groningen, The Netherlands
J. Lehmann	University of Wisconsin Hospital and Clinics, Wisconsin, U.S.A.
C. Lowther	Department of Geriatric Medicine, Royal Victoria Hospital, Edinburgh, Scotland, U.K.
M. McCarthy	Department of Community Medicine, University College London, England, U.K.
C. McKee	Department of Community Health, London School of Hygiene & Tropical Medicine, London, England, U.K.
P. Millard	Possom Controls Ltd., London, England, U.K.
G. Morasso	Department of Psychology, Istituto Tumori, Genova, Italy
M. Murphy	St. Peters Hospice, Albany, U.S.A.
H. Olesen	Clinical Psychology Department, Odense University Hospital, Odense, Denmark
A. Perakyla	Department of Sociology, University of Tampere, Tampere, Finland

A. Pointon   Hazel Grove Clinic, Stockport, England, U.K.

P. Possin   University of Wisconsin Hospital and Clinics, Wisconsin, U.S.A.

G. Rajaratnam   Department of Community Health, London School of Hygiene & Tropical Medicine, London, England, U.K.

D. Razavi   Institut Jules Bordet, Centre des Tumeurs de l'Université Libre de Bruxelles, Belgium

M. Relf   Sir Michael Sobell House, Churchill Hospital, Oxford, England, U.K.

I. Reynolds   Department of Clinical Oncology, Royal North Shore Hospital, St. Leonards, Australia

R. Richardson   Institute of Historical Research, University of London, England, U.K.

E. Robaye   Department of Psychology, Centre D'Aides aux Mourants, Bruxelles, Belgium

R. Schilling   Possum Controls Ltd., London, England, U.K.

R. Sebag-Lanoe   Geriatric Unit, Paul Brousse Hospital, Villejuif, France

R. Shapiro   Center for the Study of Bioethics, Medical College of Wisconsin, Milwaukee, U.S.A.

M. Tamburrini   Department of Psychology, Istituto Tumori, Genova, Italy

A. Urban   University of Wisconsin Hospital and Clinics, Madison, U.S.A.

M. Vachon   The Clarke Institute of Psychiatry, Toronto, Canada

A. Vainio   Department of Anaesthesiology, Helsinki University Central Hospital, Helsinki, Finland

A. Wade   Department of Community Medicine, London, England, U.K.

Communication (continued)
  with patients, 16–17, 20–21, 24–
    27, 38–39, 43–44, 59, 67
    76, 109, 114, 171, 202, 207
Community Care Team, 111, 117
Connective Unconscious, 16
Continuing Care Unit, 125
Contract funerals, 56
Coping strategies, 123, 157
Council for Music in Hospitals, 106
Counselling, 110–111, 116, 140
Cross boundary flow, 167
Cystic Fibrosis, 59, 62

Death,
  as acceptance, 6–7
    appropriate, 3, 66
    bad, 4
    best, 4–5
    better, 4–5
    catastrophic, 10
    cost-efficient, 7
    dirty, 9–10
    forbidden, 2
    good, 3–8
    good enough, 158
    healthy, 4
    honorable, 5
    horrendous, 8–10
    impersonal, 130
    normal, 8
    painful, 90
    peaceful, 90, 116
    profane, 45
    sacred, 45
    safe, 7–12
    spiteful, 7
    tamed, 32
    unsafe, 12
    vengeful, 7
    worst, 4–5
  by violence, 72
Death and fantasy, 4
Death in institutions, 66
Death Certificates, 70, 167
Death Education, 11
Death fear neurosis, 47
Death Grant, 56
Death Rates, 65, 168
Dementia, 12, 27, 29, 67, 207
Denial of death, 26
Department of Health and Social
  Security, 94–95
Depression, 66, 71–72, 156
Diamorphine, 62
Disabled Living Foundation, 97
District of Columbia, 74
Dying, 4, 6, 10, 41, 43, 63, 65,
  210
Dying child at home, 61
Dying process, 4, 48, 83

Dyspnoea, 122

Eastern and Social Services Board
  in Northern Ireland, 94
Empathy, 129
Environmental Control System, 95
Ethnographic Study of Nurses'
  Roles, 125
Euthanasia, 23, 25, 28–29, 110
Euthanatos, 126
Existential
  anxiety, 34–37
  philosophy, 33–34
  reality, 36

Factorial analyses, 175
Family coping strategies, 122
Fear of death, 48, 63
Fluid maintenance, 76
Forum of Associations, 110
Fractures, 68
Frames of death, 41–45
Frierdich's Ataxia, 95
Funerals, 53–57, 144
Funerary Nest-Egg, 53

Gastro-intestinal bleeding, 68
General model of dying process, 11
Geriatric Medicine, 68
Geriatric Units, 28–29, 68
Goal-directed symptom control, 90
Great Depression, 55
Grief, 69–73, 114, 119–123
Guilt Feelings, 41

HRCA QL Index, 71
Heart Disease, 72
Hierarchy of needs, 104
Holistic attitudes, 38
Home visiting, 72
Homeostatic mechanisms, 66
Homosexuality, 12
Hospices, 3–4, 7, 11–12, 17, 23, 28
  65, 83, 93, 96, 99, 103, 106
  110–11, 116, 130, 133–135,
  139, 142, 149, 151, 156–159
Hospices compared with traditional
  care, 6
Hospice goals, 4
Hospice Movement, 4, 11, 19–21, 109
  130
Hospice philosophy, 6, 21, 110
Hospice programs, 151–153
Huntington's Chorea, 96
Hyperalimentation, 77

Immune function, 72
Incurable acute monocytic leukemia, 43
Infective disease, 59, 61
Influenzal pneumonia, 68
Informed consent, 75

Intelligence Quotient, 191
Intensive treatment, 44
Inter-disciplinary Teams, 125-126
Inter-group rivalry, 153
Inter-role conflict, 154
Internal audit, 206
Invasive diagnostic procedures, 67
Introjection, 38
Item-total correlations, 175

JALMALV, 109, 111

Kansas Supreme Court, 75
Karnovsky Index, 207
Kidney dialysis, 76
Knowledge of one's death, 17

Lederle Laboratories, 106
Leprosy, 9
Leukemia, 43
Libido, 119
Life prolonging procedures, 76, 78
Life Satisfaction Index, 67
Life Support System, 76
Live burial, 11
Living alone, 66-67
Living Will, 75-79
Logistic regression analysis, 70
Love Story, 4
Lymphocyte function, 72

MND, 96
MST, 62
Macmillan Nurses, 133-135
Major fractures, 68
Malignant growth, 25
Marylebone, London, 56
Medical Ethics, 111
Medical Gerontological Codex, 202
Medicated survival, 110
Meningitis, 59
Minnesota Multiphasic Personality
    Inventory, 67
Model of crisis intervention,
    120-122
Morphine, 24
Motor Neurone Disease, 96
Mourning, 28, 156
Multidisciplinary Care, 24
Multidisciplinary Hospice Teams,
    99-101, 117, 125-126, 150
Multiple Handicaps, 59
Multiple incurable disease, 68
Multiple losses, 103-108
Multiple pathology, 67
Multiple pharmacy, 67
Multiple Sclerosis, 94, 96
Muscular Dystrophy, 59, 96
Muscular spasm, 61

Narcotic analgesics, 83

Naso-gastric feeding, 61
National Board of Finland, 83
National Hospice Demonstration
    Study, 6, 10
National Hospice Organisation, 126
National Hospice Study, 206
National Society for Cancer Relief, 99
Nausea, 4
Neo-natal deaths, 59
Neoplasm, 66
Nocturnal anxiety, 122
Non-verbal communication, 27
Nominal Scale, 193
Nursing Team, 125-131
Nutritional support, 76

Oblation Ritual, 29
Obstructive Airways Disease, 96
Office of Populations and Censuses
    and Surveys, 70
One-tailed 't' Test, 180
Oral antibiotic, 68
Ordini dei Medici, 193
Organ reserves, 66
Osteopetrosis, 94-95
Oxygen, 61

Pain, 4, 62, 83-84, 126
Pain control, 61, 86, 89, 93, 104,
    126
Palliative Care Unit, 109, 111, 149
Palliative treatment, 23, 25, 29,
    59, 86, 149, 155, 185
Paracetamol, 62
Paraplegic, 104
Parental support, 60
Parkinson's Disease, 96
Patient autonomy, 79
Patient and family anxiety, 155
Patients' view of dying, 6
Pauper's funeral, 55-56
Pauper's grave, 56
Pedagogical model of training, 172
Pediatric oncology, 139, 161
Pearson's Correlation Coefficient, 209
Peripheral gangrene, 68
Perforation of abdominal viscus, 68
Permitted level of anxiety, 63
Philadelphia Geriatric Morale Scale, 67
Phobia, 120
Pilgrim Hospice, 110
PLUS, 113-117
Possum Units and Systems, 94-97
Possum Trust, 95
Pre-death phase, 67
Preparatory counselling, 142
President's Commission for the Study
    of Ethical Problems in Medical
    and Biomedical and Behavioural
    Research, 72
Primal existential anxiety, 34-37